Fasting-Hydropathy-Exercise

NATURE'S WONDERFUL REMEDIES FOR THE CURE OF ALL CHRONIC AND ACUTE DISEASES

(Original Version, Restored)

by

BERNARR MACFADDEN AND FELIX OSWALD, A.M., M.D

Originally published by The Physical Culture Publishing Company, 1900

PUBLISHED BY O'Faolain Patriot L L C, Copyright 2012

info@physicalculturebooks.com

ISBN-13: 978-1481148795

ISBN-10: 1481148796

Published in the United States of America

To Order More Copies Visit: PhysicalCultureBooks.com

Health that intoxicates with its power and intensity, is within the reach of all who are willing to reason for themselves, and begin that activity of muscle, mind and body without which there can be no health, for stagnation always means disease and death.

Activity is the law of life. A machine made of the finest steel will rust and decay if not used, and the human body is not stronger than steel.

To those whose souls are rent by sorrow and pain, to those whose days and nights are heavily laden with the dull despair of physical weakness and disease, this book is respectfully dedicated.

May it be a light which guides these poor stricken human beings to the haven of perfect health, beautiful, superb—is the wish of the authors.

Awake!

Open your eyes.

Clear your brain.

Reason!

Reason clearly!

An enemy is at your door.

He has already entered nearly every home!

Is he in your home?

Are you struggling for life as he slowly

"strangles" you in his "grip of poison"?

Are your sons, your daughters, your father

or your mother fighting this fearful enemy?

If you love life, if the lives of your loved ones

are of value, begin at once to free yourself

and your home from this horrible enemy,

DRUGS.

CONTENTS

PREFACE   7

I. FASTING
I.	PHYSIOLOGICAL DATA	10
II.	THE ONE-MEAL PLAN	14
III.	DIETETIC RESTRICTIONS	23
IV.	PROTRACTED FASTS	29
V.	AN EXPERIENCE OF ONE OF THE AUTHORS IN SEVEN-DAY FAST	49

II. HYDROPATHY
VI.	PHYSIOLOGICAL DATA	58
VII.	THE COLD-WATER CURE	60
VIII.	AIR BATHS	69
IX.	CLIMATIC SANITARIA	77
X.	VENTILATION	84

III. EXERCISE
XI.	PHYSIOLOGICAL DATA	90
XII.	OUTDOOR EXERCISE	92
XIII.	INDOOR EXERCISE	98
XIV.	GYMNASTICS	104
XV.	FREE MOVEMENT CURES	114
XVI.	DETAILED ADVICE FOR TREATMENT	128

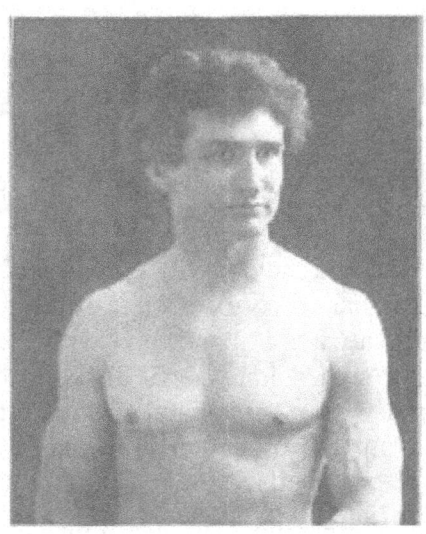

PREFACE

The great truths of Nature are here ready for you, reader.

Are you ready for them?

Are you free from prejudice, and willing to read and reason without considering the opinions of so-called authorities? To a free and intelligent human being there is no authority for him higher than his own reasoning power.

If you are free from the slavery of prejudice this book will give you food for thought. It will teach you that weakness is a crime—that it is the result of plain, easily avoided causes—that if your body is weak, or diseased, there is not the slightest excuse for remaining so—that health and strength of a high degree is the natural heritage of man and woman, and if this superb condition is not possessed, this book will clearly and concisely furnish the knowledge necessary to acquire it.

Refuse to be an invalid, reader!

Refuse to be a physical nonenity!

Are you depending upon drugs?—that gorgon horror that is torturing more human lives into misery, weakness and death than all the combined cruelties and barbarism of past ages.

Drugs! Drugs!! Great heavens, will this crime of the century never end?

Drugs never did and never will cure disease. The body cures itself if it can secure an opportunity, but with the poisonous drugs always at hand, and with their authorities standing at your side, I know it is difficult to refuse. But, friends, strengthen your minds and strike for freedom. You must be free from the drug delusion mentally before you can ever be free physically.

Years ago when my own soul was rent by the torturous belief that the health of a fully developed man was

never to be mine, I tried drugs. Nauseating and disgusting pills, powders and liquids were swallowed. The pain of my disappointment, as remedy after remedy was tried without benefit, can never be described. If I live to be a thousand years of age, there could be no experience in my life that would be stamped upon my brain quite so vividly as this.

And when freedom came at last—when the truths of Nature were revealed to me one by one, a great joy overcame me.

For I was free!

Free, friends! Free from pain, free from misery; free from weakness.

Think of it!! A freedom as glorious as the most happy moment of life!

And with this freedom came an intense desire for others to share my freedom; and drugs, the humbug, the delusion that saps your strength while they pretend to cure, will find in me a life-long enemy. As long as I have the power to think, as long as I have the power to utter a sound, my voice, my pen, my utmost energies will be expended in fighting and exposing the horrible crimes to modern humanity committed by drugs.

Read this book!!

Act upon its suggestions. Secure health with all its joy.

Be a man, complete, superb.

Or a woman, beautiful and strong.

And help me in this glorious work of stamping out the curse of weakness and disease, and the drugs that often cause this unnatural condition.

Yours for Health
Bernarr Macfadden

I - FASTING

CHAPTER I

PHYSIOLOGICAL DATA

"What shall we do to be saved?" is a question which, from a physical point of view, can be answered in less than ten words: "Learn to interpret the language of your sanitary instincts." To him who has mastered that task, the science of health is not a sealed book.

"And let me assure you, in measured words alive with conviction, that long series of cases running through seventeen years of attendance has been a line of evidence, line upon line, of the self-sufficiency of Nature to right herself in attacks of disease, no matter what the disease, or how severe its character."—E. H. Dewey, M.D.

Every living organism is a self-regulating apparatus. Our nervous system performs its functions by a combination of alarm signals that apprise us of an infinite variety of external dangers and internal needs, in a language that has a distinct expression for every want of our alimentary and respiratory organs, for every distress of our tissues, sinews and muscles, for every needed reaction against the influence of abnormal circumstances. Our skin protests against injurious degrees of heat or cold; our lungs against atmospheric impurities; our eyes against the intrusion of the smallest insect. The human body is a house that cleanses its own chambers and heats its own stoves, opens and shuts its windows at proper intervals, expels mischievous intruders and promptly informs its tenant of every external peril and internal disorder.

If it were not for the perverting influence of baneful sanitary superstitions we should run no risk of mistaking poison for food, nor of substituting unnatural for natural stimulants. We should never have conceived the idea that the sick must be forced to swallow virulent drugs; all our "ailments and pains, in form, variety and degree beyond description," could be cured by the three remedies of Nature: Exercise, fasting and refrigeration.

The application of those remedies is not followed by distressing after effects. It does not develop a morbid hankering for a repetition of the prescription in constantly increasing doses.

Compare the effects of outdoor exercise with those of Dr. Quack's Digestion Bitters, as characteristic instances of normal and abnormal tonics. Both prescriptions tend to stimulate the appetite. But how? And at what expense? To the palate of a healthy child alcohol is almost as repulsive as corrosive sublimate: Nature's protest against the incipience of a health-destroying habit. Nor does instinct yield to the first disregard of its appeals: Nausea, gripes, nervous headaches and gastric spasms warn the novice again and again. But we repeat the dose, and Nature, true to her highest law of preserving existence at any price, and realizing the hopelessness of the life-endangering struggle, finally chooses the alternative of palliating an evil for which she has no remedy, and adapts herself to the abnormal condition. "The body of the dram-drinker," says a medical reformer, "becomes a poison-engine, an alcohol-machine, performing its vital functions only under the spur of a specific stimulus. And only then the unnatural habit begets that craving which the toper comes to mistake for the prompting of a healthy appetite—a craving which every gratification makes more exorbitant. For by and by the jaded system fails to respond to the spur; the poison-slave has to resort to stronger stimulants.

And, moreover, every excitation of the flagging vital energies is followed by a debilitating reaction. The bowels fail to act; disinclination to physical and mental efforts makes work a penalty. The "pleasant and exhilarating tonic "has evolved the soul-darkening mists of Katzenjammer. As a net result of his experiment Dr. Quack's customer finds himself worse than before by just as much as the unnatural stimulant has still further exhausted his small reserve fund of vital vigor.

The benefits of the movement cure, on the other hand, are not heralded by the kettledrum methods of Quackstetter & Co.; but they can dispense with such endorsements. Outdoor sports commend themselves to the instincts of a healthy child as unmistakably as wholesome food and pure air. Exercise creates an expenditure of energy that has to be replaced by stimulating the functions of every organ; effete tissues are eliminated; the heart beats stronger and faster, the lungs, liver and kidneys respond to the spur; the whole system works as a machine under an increase of steam-pressure. The same healthy, prompt and harmless tonic reacts upon the bowels; the problem of digestive stimulation has been solved without the risk of distressing after-effects. No baneful habit has fastened upon the patient; no drastic suppression of symptoms has made the remedy worse than the evil. The disorder has been cured by the removal of its cause. And all these advantages can be claimed for the Fasting Cure.

"Take away food from a sick man's stomach and you have begun, not to starve the sick man, but the disease."— E. H. Dewey, M.D.

"The principle on which the fasting-cure acts is one on which all physiologists agree, and one which is readily explained and understood. We know that in animal life the law of nature is for the effete, worn out, and least vitalized matter to be first cast off. We see this upon the cuticle, nails, hair, and in the snake the casting off of his old skin. Now in wasting or famishing from the want of food, this process of elimination goes on in a much more rapid manner than ordinarily, and the vital force, which would otherwise be expended in digesting the food taken, acts now in expelling from the vital domain, whatever morbid matters it may contain. This, then, is a beautiful idea in regard to the fasting-cure—that whenever a meal of food is omitted, the body purifies itself thus much from its disease, and this becomes apparent in the subsequent amendment, both as regards bodily feeling and strength. It is proved, also, in the fact that during the prevalence of epidemics, those who have been obliged to live almost in a state of starvation, have gone free from an attack, while the well-fed have been cut off in numbers by the merciless disease."—Joel Shaw, M.D.

CHAPTER II

THE ONE-MEAL PLAN

The progress of culture often resembles the undulating rise of the tide, rather than the steady advance of a river current; the rippling waves surge in capricious eddies and for a time may even seem to recede. Scientific tenets familiar to the philosophers of pagan antiquity were lost sight of during the night of the Middle Ages, and in the dawn of modern civilization are apt to be viewed with doubt or accepted as novel discoveries.

The true theory of the solar system, for instance, was known to the disciples of Pythagoras; but a thousand years later was forgotten almost as completely as the existence of the lost Atlantis. Centuries before the birth of Ludwig Jahn the Greeks had recognized the truth that in thickly settled countries the lack of wood-sports ought to be compensated by gymnastic training and competitive athletics. There were fresh-air doctors two thousand years before Dio Lewis, and during the zenith period of Grecian and Roman civilization monogamy was not half as firmly established as the rule that a health-loving man should content himself with one meal a day, and never eat till he had leisure to digest, i. e., not till the day's work was wholly done.

For more than a thousand years the one meal plan was the established rule among the civilized nations inhabiting the coast-lands of the Mediterranean. The evening repast—call it supper or dinner—was a kind of domestic festival, the reward of the day's toil, an enjoyment which rich and poor refrained from marring by premature gratifications of their appetite. Cares were laid aside before the family and their guests assembled in the supper-hall. People of wealth provided reclining couches, and their desserts included a good many things besides Attic figs. They treated their guests to perfumes, to music and dances. Athensus describes a symposium enlivened by musical contests and juggler shows. All but the poorest had at least a minstrel who bartered comic ditties for a basketful of cold lunch. Amusements of that sort were supposed to aid digestion and keep the revelers awake during the two hours' interval between the termination of the repast and the setting of the sun, though appetite alone generally guaranteed the assimilation of a good-sized meal. Dinner, in the form of a noon-time lunch was unknown, and for breakfast a biscuit or a piece of crust, to counteract the acidity of the stomach, were considered sufficient.

There were exceptions, but they were tolerated merely as we should tolerate a sportsman unable to wait for legal holidays, and enjoying leisure periods in the middle of the week, or vacations before the beginning of summer. "To desecrate one's appetite," the Romans called the habit of eating between meals, and Suetonius mentions among the demerits of the Emperor Vitellius a "penchant for gorging himself in the early morning hours,"—the time of the day that ought to have remained consecrated to labor or study. As a rule, probably nine out of ten well-educated Greeks and six out of ten Romans did not think twenty-two hours too long an interval between meals which, with chat and other pauses, lasted more than an hour and a half.

"They were probably athletes," remarked a critic of a lecture on Roman customs; "but what about women and persons of delicate constitutions? Would they not risk to faint with hunger in trying total abstinence, in that extreme sense of the word, all the day long?"

In reply to such questions the lecturer ought to have added a few words on the subject of Diet and the Influence of Habit. A little child, according to Dr. Page's experiments, can be taught to guzzle day and night, or to content himself with being stilled about once in three hours. Little habitues of a hundred daily guzzles will howl horribly at the first attempt to restrict them to seventy-five, but after a month or two will get so used to ten nursings that it requires coaxing to make them accept a dozen.

And in the course of a few years the tapering-off process can be easily brought to an average of one meal a day. Baker Pasha (Sir Samuel Baker) ascertained that fact in studying the habits of the Abyssinian hunters. Youngsters of twelve years join the hunting expeditions of their tribe and think themselves lucky if the kettle can be set a-boiling to the extent of furnishing a good evening meal. In the repose of the kraal they might yield to the temptation of a noon-time lunch; but when game is scarce, think nothing of rolling themselves up in a blanket at night and trying a nap to forget the disappointment of the day, trusting to the chance of better pot-luck for the morrow. "Qui dort dine," say the French—"he who sleeps feasts." A good night's rest in the bracing night air of the Abyssinian tablelands will sustain strength even on the basis of alternate day meals. A daily feast is so abundantly sufficient that active youngsters would fear to handicap themselves by re-loading their stomachs before the end of the next day. With the prospect of an up-and-down hill race against time and the competition of athletic companions, the offer even of a moderate morning lunch would probably jar upon their sanitary conscience.

The subjects of the two Kaisers, on the other hand, would consider it a grievance to be limited to three daily meals. All over Germany and northern Austria a pause of four hours is thought a distressingly long time between meals, though some brands of wurst are apt to resist the assimilative apparatus of unfeathered bipeds at least half a clay.

Master Karl Schulze has no springboks to hunt; the stifling atmosphere of his grammar-school room does not promote digestion; yet Karl insists on a Fruhstuck (breakfast) six A.

M.; zweites frustuck ("second breakfast") at nine; mittagsmahl at noon; vesperbrot (vesper lunch) at half past three; and abendessen at 6 P. M. Just before retiring from the scene of their gastronomic exploits Vienna burghers often add a night-cap of beer, pretzels and more wurst, "for the stomach's sake." "In spite of the stomach" might seem more correct, but it isn't. One month's practice would be enough to supplement the horrid load of ingesta with a midnight meal. It might shorten the glutton's life one half; but as sure as the noon and night comes around his stomach, or the ulcerated receptacle retaining that name, would interrupt the nightmare circus to clamor for its perquisites; and disappointment would result in fits of insomnia and yearnings for the picnic grounds of a better hereafter.

It is the same with fluid surfeits. Hoffs Malt Extract was advertised as a cure-all till even ascetics bought a bottle at certain times of the year—say a quart per quarter, and on those terms contrived to compromise with the stimulant habit. After the end of the second month they might now and then experience a vague yearning for the office of the Hoff Agency, but on the whole get along contentedly without half way drinks. In Munich almost identical beverages have votaries that get nervous if business emergencies oblige them to postpone their trip to the Bier-Keller for a few minutes. They call thrice a day, and after supper hurry to a club that furnishes them a pretext for guzzling till midnight. "Say, I feel a vacuum," one of these far-gones used to remark, when the Sunday excursion steamer did not reach its pier strictly on time. Nay, a Wisconsin physician vouches for the fact that some of the Milwaukee brewers allow their employees twenty-five quarts of lager free, every working day in the year, and that many of the veterans begin to fret if they cannot visit the free dispensary at least once in thirty minutes. Habit, in fact, becomes a "second nature," and the limits of its influence, for better or worse, have never been ascertained. It is quite possible that gluttons might learn to hanker for a meal an hour, and that St. Jerome in his Syrian hermitage really got along comfortably with three meals a week; but it must be admitted that the old Roman plan combines advantages not easy to rival.

Like a festival at the end of the week, it sustains the energy of the laborer with the prospect of an adequate reward. The gratification of a well-earned appetite is something very different from the listless compliance with a conventional custom or the attendance at a regulation meal which a sanitary intuition denounces as an aggravation of an already grievous surfeit. A twenty-two hours' fast will make a meal of bread and baked apples more palatable than all the arts of the Freres Provenceaux could make three daily banquets to a dyspeptic.

One great advantage of frequent meals is founded on the fact that repletion does not at once announce itself to the instinct of a gormand, and that the interval preceding a decided consciousness of satiety may have been abused for a congestion of the alimentary system. Upon the one-meal plan that risk is obviated, or at least greatly lessened. After a fast of twenty-two hours it is almost impossible to eat with relish more than the system can utilize in the course of a night and a day.

The Roman custom also obviated an affliction that has turned thousands of plow-boys into tramps and driven more than one dyspeptic to suicide, viz.: the misery of hard work directly after a full meal. "I didn't mind being waked before daybreak to feed the cows," says a rural correspondent of the Chautauquan. "I could stand wood-chopping in a sleet-storm and ditching in an all-day drizzle, but if the old man routed me out of my siesta nap under the canopy of a shade tree to recommence plowing in the blazing sun, I felt things that can be only summarized in the impression that the change from wigwams to modern farms was a mistake, if the attainment of happiness has anything to do with the purposes of civilization."

And those protests of instinct are, indeed, well founded. Not only that the progress of digestion is thus interrupted, not only that the body derives no strength from the inert mass of ingesta, but that mass, by undergoing a putrid instead of peptic decomposition, vitiates the humors of the system it was intended to nourish, irritates the sensitive membranes of the stomach, and gradually impairs the vigor of the whole digestive apparatus.

"Plenus renter non studet libenter," was a Latin proverb— "a filled stomach abhors study," and immediately after dinner mental efforts are certainly quite as ill-timed as hard bodily labor. No other hygienic mistake, not even the stimulant fallacy, has done so much to make ours a generation of dyspeptics. Brain-work interferes with digestion as noise and motion interfere with sleep. Hence, the sallow complexion, the hollow eyes, and the weary gait of thousands of city clerks, scholars, lawyers, newspaper hacks, and even physicians. Hence, the gastric torments of poor, overworked teachers, who (unlike happier servants of the public) cannot shirk their work, and have to snatch their dinner during a brief interval of the hardest kind of mental drudgery.

The evening-dinner plan would obviate all that misery. The noon-recess could be devoted to a bath, a half hour's chat in the shade, and the toiler would return to his work refreshed. That contrast, once known from practical experience, would preclude the temptation of a return to the unsanitary plan. Boys in their early teens can be taught to consider eating between evening meals a transgression against the health-laws of Nature. Dr. J. H. Lincoln of Hamilton County, Tennessee, had trained his youngsters in rational dietetics till he could trust them not to break their noonday fast for the sake of any tidbits. "For shame!" he used to say, "the idea of wanting to eat before your day's work is done! It's just as if a mechanic should claim his wages before he had earned them."

Evening diners also escape the risk of sunstrokes. "Surfeit strokes" would be a far more appropriate name for an affection almost unknown in Spanish America, where rich and poor suspend labor during the heat of the afternoon. The self-regulating tendency of our organism can hold its own against a temperature of 105 degrees Fahrenheit in the shade; it might resist the added grievance of superfluous clothing, but succumbs to a combination of sun-heat, sweltering dry-goods, and superheated, greasy made-dishes. A sunstroke fit is, in fact, caused by what physicians call a "zymotic process of blood-changes"—in plainer words, the humors of the living body begin to ferment. The system has ways of its own to counteract that risk, but may try in vain to apply them when its energies are diverted by the task of compromising a reckless surfeit. Who has not noticed the bodily and mental vigor that facilitates all sorts of work in the early morning hours? It is only partly due to a difference of temperature, for indoor-workers, too, experience its benefits, and it would be a mistake to suppose that the invigorating effects of a good night's rest are limited to the early forenoon. At least half the morning energy is due to the fact that exemption from the task of digestion makes the reserve stores of vital vigor available for other work. The first meal forfeits that advantage, and by the simple plan of postponing breakfast the buoyancy of the early morning hours can be enjoyed all day.

"My body is all forehead," said the naked Indian, when his Caucasian hunting companion wondered that he did not shiver in a snow-storm: and the faster's day is all morning.

If you cannot adopt the one-meal plan at once at least avoid breakfast. Here is how Dr. Dewey describes his first forenoon without breakfast:

"I had a forenoon of such lofty mental cheer, such energy of soul and body, such a sense of physical ease as I had not known since a young man in my later teens. When the dinner-hour came there was an added relish that was a new experience, and I left the table with a stomach so supplied that there was no need of apprehension as to an attack of faintness during the afternoon. There is no natural hunger in the morning after a night of restful sleep, because there has been no such degree of cell destruction as to create a demand for food at the ordinary hour of the American breakfast. Sleep is not a hunger-causing process. To reinforce this statement and the reasons behind it, is the experience of thousands who have abandoned the morning meal, and in a short time lost all hint of a need of it. This could not have been had there been a need, for Nature is imperious, exacting; and it is not in the line of possibility that she will permit any getting used to less food than she requires to preserve her physiological balance. She easily permits you to skip that meal you do not need so soon after the refreshing sleep and which you always eat from habit; but later she will call you to account if you give less than her demands.

"Now you are to abolish your breakfast, and not to presume to eat again without keen hunger; this hunger you may have if you wait for it, even while sitting in an arm chair, or lying in bed, and it will be for food as nourishing as the axman requires. What shall be eaten at each meal will be a law for self to determine. No food is good or healthful, and therefore typical, without a special demand for it. Keen hunger, the most relishing of foods, thoroughly masticated, a recreative state of mind during digestion, these are the easily acquired conditions behind sustained health.

"But how sudden the revelation to me! Go without your breakfast and you will be hungry for your dinner ! And so hungry that you will forget to take your cod-liver dose!

And the dinner is so well relished, and you feel so much better after it that you conclude to omit the dosing altogether! How simple! Only to fast, no matter if it costs a whole day, a whole week, or a whole month, and with absolute safety; why, do you not recall how energetically the digestive organs will work over the keenly relished food after the long fast due to fevers? How much more, then, may be expected from fasts that are to be no tax on vital power? Safe? Yes, beyond any question. As soon as the stomach and appendages have disposed of the decomposing, unbidden meals that are still a tax on vital power, there will be a positive increase of mental and physical power, so that when Nature's own signal for food is given, there is none of the exhausted feeling that is more or less realized before the needless morning meal.

"Appetite will always come where death is not inevitable, no less in the ordinary conditions of low health than in cases of acute sickness, and fasting is the swiftest, the most effectual and the most unfailing of all devices ever conceived for inviting natural hunger. Keen hunger, hunger only, makes known the individual need."

CHAPTER III

DIETETIC RESTRICTIONS

A "fast," in the language of the medieval churchmen, generally implied the interdiction of special kinds of food, and, in that sense of the word, almost every creed of ancient and modern times prescribes periods of total abstinence. The Rhamadan, or Lenten season, of the Mohammedans, has to be observed for a couple of months, though the casuists of the Koran allow travelers and busy laborers to shorten the term by lengthening the list of forbidden viands. The successors of Joe Smith prohibit alcoholic stimulants to all but invalids, and Zoroaster interdicts wine and "soma-juice"—probably some opiate— to those who can procure more wholesome tonics.

The Pythagoreans went further and tabooed wine altogether. Strict followers of the sect (whose "philosophy" was to all purposes a religion) abstained also from flesh food and, for some never wholly explained reason, from beans. Peter Bayle surmised some figurative significance of that tenet— beans of various colors being used for political ballots, but Pliny distinctly states that the mere touch of the plant was considered a defilement, and that in the war against Sybaris a squad of orthodox Pythagoreans allowed themselves to be cut to pieces, rather than seek safety in a bean-field.

That doctrine would not have flourished in Boston, though its apostle enjoyed the reputation of a Trismeglstus— a past-master of wisdom, and was supposed to have entered Olympus by some gate closed to mortals of ordinary intelligence.

Both the Buddhists and Brahmans enjoin total abstinence from flesh-food, and Sir William Jones attests the fact that starving Hindus "declined to save their lives by sacrificing those of their dumb fellow-creatures."

In all those cases the interdict had a moral significance. Wine clouds the mind that should seek to obtain glimpses of a brighter world. Flesh food stimulates the animal passions, and certainly excites combativeness. A diet of bull beef imbued our North American Redskins with the ferocity of carnivorous beasts, while their banana- eating kinsmen of Southern Mexico are as placid as Hindus.

But a large number of dietetic restrictions might be recommended from a purely physical point of view. Alcohol is a liver-poison and aggravates the virulence of many diseases so unmistakably that its victims have hardly a right to complain of chronic disorders. Theirs are ailments perpetuated by a chronic provocation of the cause, and not apt to appeal to the sympathy of total abstainers any more than the afflictions of trichinosis could evoke the fears of a pork-abhoring Jew.

Drunkards, it is true, plead their "willingness to reform if the flesh were not stronger than the spirit." Temperance preachers descant on the dangers of worldly temptations and selfish indulgences, or the lusts of unregenerate hearts as if our natural appetites were tempting us to our ruin. Nay, the stimulant vice has found learned defenders; the followers of Paracelsus have worshiped the man-devouring fire as a sacred flame; for thousands of honest truth-seekers the disagreement of doctors makes it doubtful if alcohol is a friend or a foe, a health-giving tonic or a death-dealing poison. Is that uncertainty not a proof that in one most important respect Nature has failed to insure the welfare of her creatures?

What it really proves is this: That habitual sin has blunted our physical conscience till we have not only ceased to heed, but ceased to understand, the protests of our inner monitor. It proves that the victims of vice have so utterly forgotten the language of their instincts that they are no longer able to distinguish a natural appetite from a morbid appetency.

For it might be questioned if the instinctive horror of carrion is stronger than a normal man's aversion to the first taste of alcohol. To the palate of an unseduced youngster brandy is intensely repulsive, lager beer as nauseous as sewer swill; wine is simply spoiled musk, as unattractive as acidulated sugar-water. Is it Nature's fault that these health-protecting instincts can be perverted by a deliberate and ever-repeated disregard of their warning? Or can flesh-gluttons ("corpse-eaters" the editor of the Vegetarian calls them) plead the weakness of Nature, the lures of the flesh and the devil?"

Without spices and kitchen tricks animal food would not tempt the progeny of Adam to any damaging extent. "If I didn't want people to eat my apples I wouldn't lock them up in my orchard," says an irreverent critic of Genesis; but I do believe that an unperverted child could be locked up with a couple of helpless lambs, and that, like Sir William's Hindus, it would lie down and die, sooner than save its life by sacrificing that of its dumb fellow- creatures. For, quite aside from moral scruples, the protests of instinct would prevent. Starvation—hunger intensified to the degree of fearful torture—would fail to overcome the natural aversion to the taste of raw (i.e., undisguised) flesh food.

And cooking cannot destroy all the disease-germs which the "corpse-eater" transfers to his own body. The task of assimilating wolf-food is an affront to our digestive organs. Our stomachs, bowels, and teeth are those of a fruit- eating creature.

"Don't you think there is something objectionable about a draughty bedroom window in this changeable climate of ours?" a Connecticut foggy asked Dio Lewis.

"That's just my opinion," said the facetious doctor; "in ninety-nine out of a hundred cases the draught isn't near strong enough."

And the main objection to ecclesiastic fasts is the circumstance that they were rarely persistent enough. "Fasting," i.e., abstaining from meat on Friday and for a few weeks in early spring can hardly be expected to undo the mischief of two hundred and seventy-five carnivorous days.

Our instinct-guided Darwinian kinsmen are frugal in the original sense of the word; i.e., subsist chiefly on tree- fruit, but have no objection to eggs, and vegetarians of the Alcott school may have prejudiced their cause by prohibiting eggs, milk, and all kinds of fat, as well as meat.

But in midsummer it would certainly often be a good plan to stick to an Alcott menu for a few weeks. Faire mai- gre (literally, "make lean") the French call fasting, but adopt their Lenten fare at the wrong time of the year. The idea of insisting on three daily meals of greasy, apopleptic, heat-aggravating viands is preposterous at a season that makes the struggle for existence a fight against a fever-heat atmosphere; nor is there any real need for "something warm" three times a day. We might as well aggravate the grievance of a blizzard with artificial refrigerants, or swallow opiates while imploring heaven for strength to watch and pray. Perpetual Lents, modified by an occasional omelette, are not incompatible with perfect comfort, and total abstainer from stimulants should sign a pledge against tea and coffee, while they are about it.

Only unnatural appetencies have no natural limits, and a combination of dietetic restrictions with the one-meal plan would enable us to dispense with, the sickening cant of the saints who ask us to make our dinners as many ordeals for the exercise of self-denial. "It would justify suicide," says an educational reformer, "if this world of ours were really arranged on the diabolic plan of making every gratification of our natural instincts injurious."

"Stop eating whenever the taste of a special dish tempts you to unusual indulgence." . . . "In saying grace, add in silence a pledge to prove your self-control;" "test the superiority of moral principles to physical appetites," and similar apothegms recall the time when moralists tried to earn heaven by trampling the strawberry patches of earth and obtain forgiveness for eating at all by mixing their food with a decoction of wormwood. "Stop eating when you relish your food more than usually?" Nego et pernego! We might as well tell a health-seeker to refrain from sleep when he feels specially drowsy.

"Regulate the quality of your meals and let the quantity take care of itself," is a far more sensible rule. Wholesome food rarely tempts us to indulge to excess. We do not often hear of milk topers or baked-apple gluttons.

"Do not eat till you have leisure to digest," but after a fast-day, and with all night for digestion and assimilation, do not insult Nature by being afraid to eat your fill of wholesome food. If a combination of exceptional circumstances should, nevertheless, result in a surfeit, do not rush to the shop of the bluepill vender, but try the effect of a longer fast.

"Every disease that afflicts mankind is a constitutional possibility developed into disease by more or less habitual eating in excess of the supply of gastric juices!

"The sense of taste then, you see, as you have not quite realized before, exists for a two-fold purpose, (1.) To indicate the precise food needed to restore the wastes of muscle energy, and (2.) that there shall be no mistakes made, the needed food is to be the most keenly relished. Now with this to guide you hereafter you will not need to study the science of food analysis, if you so allow your appetite to develop that Nature can order the bill of fare out loud with the clearest enunciation."—E. H. Dewey, M.D.

CHAPTER IV
PROTRACTED FASTS

The strongest temperance argument I ever heard was the incidental remark of a lecturing naturalist, that "it would be easy to name a thousand different animals that subsist on a thousand different kinds of food, but that they all drink water."

The question as to the most effective and most natural remedy might be settled with similar conclusiveness. Crapulent dogs can now and then be seen eating grass, and after a surfeit of green fodder ruminants evince a hankering after salt, but serious sickness prompts all animals to fast. Wounded deer will retire to some secluded glen and starve for weeks together. In the southern Alleghanies, where mineral efflorescences, mingling with stagnant water cause a disorder known as "milk sickness," the animals thus affected get "off their feed," and by rest and total abstinence generally contrive to recover without medical assistance in the course of a week or two.

A fortnight's fast does not preclude the hope of survival. In the moulting season certain cage birds prefer to get along for a month with a minimum of food, to compensate the lack of facilities for active exercise, and I remember the case of a little dachshund (a species of bowlegged terrier) that survived a fall from the loft of a tall building by three weeks of almost total abstinence. During a visit to the riding-school of a cavalry regiment I had turned over the little waddler to a sergeant, who put him in a barn, and finding that he could crawl out under the gate and was apt to come to grief by being kicked by a horse, finally put him in a bag and ordered one of the men to lock him up in the hay-loft at the top of the building. That checked his restlessness for the time being, but on stepping out on the street, an hour after, I heard a whine as from the clouds, and looking up saw my dachshund crouching on the edge of an open louvre and yelping crescendo, to draw my attention to the discomfiture of his situation. In the next moment he had lost his balance, and after a series of aerial somersaults, landed on the hard pavement, with a crack that seemed to have broken every bone in his body. Blood was trickling from his mouth and nostrils when they picked him up, and the troopers advised me to "put him out of misery," but he was my little brother's pet, and, after some hesitation, I decided to take him home in a basket and give the problem of his cure the benefit of a fractional chance. Investigation proved that he had broken two legs and three ribs, and judging by the way he raised his head and gasped for air, every now and then, it seemed probable that his lungs had been injured.

The location of his grave had already been settled; but the next morning he was still alive and lapped up a pint of water. For twenty days and twenty nights the little terrier stuck to life and his cotton-lined basket, without touching a crumb of solid food, but ever ready to lick up a few drops of cold water, in preference even to milk or soup. At the end of the third week he made an effort to leave his couch, and a few days after contrived to stagger along the floor to get the benefit of a hearth-fire. He had broken his fast with a saucerful of sweet milk, but only on the evening of the twenty-sixth day began to betray a personal interest in the contents of a plateful of meat-scraps that had been placed near his basket every morning.

Before the end of the winter he accompanied his friends to that same riding-school and was introduced to the veterinary surgeon of the regiment. Misknit bones had made his crooked legs a trifle crookeder, but he could run again and attest the vigor of his lungs by a lusty bark. A clear case of recovery in spite of—we did not venture to say because of—total abstinence from drugs.

"What did you feed him on?" inquired the surgeon, taking it for granted that Nature must have been assisted somehow or other.

"Nothing, for the first three weeks."

"What?"

"Nothing, sir. Or, to be quite exact, nothing except some air and water."

The surgeon shook his head. "Stout chaps, these daxes," he muttered, caressing the paradox with the tip of his boot. "The vitality of those brutes!" he probably thought to himself; "the idea of that thing recovering in spite of such neglect."

Surgeon K. had a horseload of instruments and might have succeeded in dosing the patient with a prescription of beef, wine and iron, by means of a stomach-funnel. If the little dachshund could have survived the additional affliction, is another question.

The fasting-cure instinct is not limited to our dumb fellow-creatures. It is a common experience that pain, fevers, gastric congestions, and even mental afflictions take away the appetite," and only unwise nurses will try to thwart the purpose of Nature in that respect. The manager of a large Michigan sanitarium makes it a rule to let his attendants indulge his patients with all the cold water they want to drink, or even coax them to try another glass, but never urge them to eat against their inclination.

"Abstinence is by far too much feared in the treatment of acute diseases generally. We have good reason for believing that many a life has been destroyed by the indiscriminate feeding which is so often practised among the sick. The safety of abstinence will be apparent when we remember how often persons have lain in fevers, dysentery, and other prostrating diseases, fourteen, twenty-one, and even more days without nutriment, and in the end doing well."—Joel Shaw. M.D.

The "Health-school of Talerno," in its "Vade-mecum of Sanitary Maxims," has an apothegm to the effect that "The more you feed a sick body the sicker you make it," and Dr. Isaac Jennings, the author of "Medical Reform," expresses the same truth in an emphatic manner of his own. "Don't aggravate the troubles of a sick fellow-man," he says, "by forcing him to swallow food against the protest of his stomach.

"No one ever thinks of eating if the appetite is abolished by a trivial ailment and plainly for the reason that it would be an unpleasant experience attended by depressing results; but if the ailment is thought dangerous, why, then the physics and chemistry of digestion are utterly ignored, and food must be enforced.

"There is a very general concurrence of opinion that the aversion to food that characterizes all cases of acute disease, which is fully in proportion to the severity of the symptoms, is one of Nature's blunders that requires the intervention of art, and hence enforced feeding regardless of aversion.

"I can have no doubt that feeding during illness when no hunger exists is a disease-prolonging agency.

"The more I study the question of nutrition in disease at the bedside of acute illness the more am I unable to comprehend the logic of giving the sick, and especially the very sick, a form of food that even in the most vigorous health cannot be borne, even for a single day, without a lowering of vital power; nay, that where even one meal of it cannot be put into the stomach of hunger without a clearly perceptible loss of power.

"No physician will admit that normal health can be maintained for a single day, for the above reasons, on milk and whisky; then where is the logic of feeding it to the sick? How expect, by its use, to raise abnormal health to the normal, when it inevitably lowers the normal to the abnormal?

"Most of the need of drugs to allay restlessness or pain, and to enforce sleep in cases of the severely sick, arises from the exhaustive taxing of the vital power from the enforced feeding and stimulation."—E. H. Dewey, M.D.

There is no danger in temporary abstinence. Nature knows best. . . . Accustom yourself in all your little ailments, and also in your grave and more distressing affections, to regard the movement concerned in them in a friendly aspect— designed for and tending to the removal of a difficulty of whose existence you were unaware, and which, if suffered to remain and accumulate, might prove the destruction of the house you live in. And that, instead of its symptoms needing to be suppressed, they are themselves curative operations, and that what should be called the disease, lies back of them, as the real disorder or difficulty which they are intended to remove."

The physiological rationale of the fasting instinct is this: The task of digestion monopolizes the vital energies of the organism to a degree that interferes with emergency work. While the kitchen is undergoing repairs to undo the mischief of a storm or a conflagration, the cook would ask to be excused from routine drudgery. No care could obviate the risk of her fritters getting sprinkled with plaster-dust or showers of soot, and pending renovation she would expect her folks to shift with cold lunch, preserves, and other winter-stores of the pantry. Even thus Nature tries to remove the obstacles of a remedial problem. When mustering her energies for a struggle with a critical disorder she prefers to be exempted from other work, and, as it were, get her hands free for the effective and rapid accomplishment of a task that may admit of no delay. The functions of the alimentary organs are thus temporarily suspended. Lack of appetite, or even a violent aversion to food, are physiological intimations of the fact that the kitchen-department of the organism has been closed for repairs. But that arrangement implies no risk of starvations.

"When death occurs before the skeleton condition is reached it is always due to old age or some form of disease or injury, and not to starvation."—E. H. Dewey, M.D.

There are alimentary reserve stores; accumulations of adipose tissue gathered to guard against this. They will supply all essential needs for the time being, and can be replaced at leisure, after the work of reconstruction has been finished. In some cases they may have been put away for the needs of old age, but are now drawn upon for a transient emergency. The body, so to say, has for a time to make shift with its winter stores.

These nutritive reserves are ready for use at short notice and their application to the momentary needs of the system does not interfere with other work. Digestive problems, in other senses of the word, would prove a serious handicap upon the efficacy of the disease fighters, and, moreover, could be solved only in a perfunctory manner. The ingesta would have to be concocted and hurried out without real benefit to the department of nutrition.

In the case of mental affections that precaution has sometimes a peculiar by-purpose. Care, worry, but especially fits of rage, have a tendency to vitiate the humors of the system, and precautionary Nature shuts off the kitchen- supplies to prevent more serious mischief.

Dr. Carpenter in his "Mental Physiology," quotes the experience of an Austrian doctor who was called to the death-bed of a child poisoned by the milk of its own mother. A soldier had been quartered in the house, and one day came in drunk and promptly picked a quarrel with the paterfamilias—a poor Bohemian shoemaker. A scuffle followed, the drunken ruffian drew his sword and the cobbler was getting worsted, when suddenly his wife rushed in and with the superhuman strength of fury overpowered the intruder, snatched his sword and snapped it into pieces. Neighbors interposed, and the cobbler's wife, still trembling with excitement, sat down to nurse her baby. A few minutes after, the child began to twist as in a fever fit, and died in convulsions, though medical assistance had been instantly summoned.

It has also been noticed that the bite of tortured animals often becomes poisonous. In a last resort of self-defence the organism has evolved an avenging virus, but observes the precaution to cut off the appetite for food, in order to lessen the risk of the envenomed saliva entering the circulation and its blood-poison reaching the wrong address.

More or less every disorder of the organic function involves a risk of food turning into poison, and thus suggests a secondary significance of the fasting instinct.

In other words, food, eaten in the crisis of a serious disease, would not only hamper the work of cure, but might expose the system to an added peril.

Over-eating has become a vice of enormous prevalence, and for millions a protracted fast would prove a specific for the cure of ailments that defy medication. Diarrhoea, for instance, admits of no readier or more harmless remedy. It is a result of dietetic abuses and Nature's usual way to evacuate irritant substances—often accumulations of indigestible food threatening to become virulent under the influence of a high temperature.

A day's fast would mitigate the trouble. Two days of total abstinence would generally cure it and leave the condition of the alimentary organs improved in every way. But the patient cannot wait. Instead of earning the right to health he wants to buy it ready-made over the counter, and applies to a drug-monger. Loose bowels indicate a deficiency of vital strength, yet nearly every debilitating poison of the vegetable and mineral kingdom has been employed to paralyze the activity, and, as it were, silence the protest of the rebellious organs. Bismuth, arsenic, calomel, opium, mercury, nux vomica, zinc salts, acetate of lead and nitrate of silver are among the gentle "aids to Nature" that have been prescribed to control the revolt of the mutinous bowels. An attempt to control a fit of vomiting by choking the neck of the patient would be an analogous mistake. The prescription operates as long as the vitality of the bowels is absolutely paralyzed by the virulence of the drug; but the first return of functional energy will be used to eject the poison.

That new protest is silenced by the same argument; for awhile the exhaustion of the whole system is mistaken for a sign of submission, till a fresh revolt calls for a repetition of the coercive measures. In the meantime the organism suffers under a compound system of starvation; the humors are surcharged with virulent matter, the whole digestive apparatus withdraws its aid from the needs of the vital economy, and the flame of life feeds on the store of tissue; the patient wastes far more rapidly than an unpoisoned person would on an air-and-water diet.

It is not too much to say that the timely application of the fasting cure would have saved such patients nine-tenths of their time and trouble. Denutrition, or the temporary deprivation of food, exercises an astringent influence as part of its general conservative effect. The organism, stinted in its supply of vital resources, soon begins to curtail its current expenditure. The movements of the respiratory process decrease; the temperature of the body sinks; the secretion of bile and uric acid is diminished, and before long the retrenchment of the assimilative functions reacts on the intestinal organs; the colon contracts and the smaller intestines retain all but the most irritating ingesta.

A persistent hunger-cure will eliminate even an active virus by a gradual molecular catalysis and removal of the inorganic elements. No deepest-seated microbes have a living chance against that method of expurgation. With no digestive drudgery on hand, Nature employs the long-desired leisure for general house-cleaning purposes. The accumulations of superfluous tissue are overhauled and analyzed; the available component parts to be turned over to the department of nutrition, the refuse to be thoroughly and permanently removed. Germ diseases are swept out together with other rubbish. Influenza (La Grippe) can be nipped in the bud by a few days of total abstinence. Its microbes are preparing to feed on pulmonary tissues, but are bundled out before they have time to entrench their position. Catarrh ("colds") and incipient consumption can be cured in the same manner, and a U. S. army surgeon reports the case of a patient wrecked on the coast of southern Texas and reaching civilization only after a month of dreadful hardships, that reduced him to a living skeleton, but permanently cured his lung disorder. The mystery of the "King's Evil" cures probably admits of a similar solution. At a time when scrofula was ten times more prevalent than nowadays, thousands of health-seekers crowded the ante-chambers of royal palaces, to be touched by the hand of an anointed king. The Lord's anointed was in many cases a worn-out rake with his own hide full of germ- diseases, but his touch rarely missed its effect on patients who had come from a considerable distance, whence Dr. Burnett's remark that the natives of farthest Scotland and Ireland trusted the miraculous power of their sovereign more than his next neighbors. Scrofulous cockneys, who could reach the royal presence by crossing the street, crossed in vain; but pilgrims who had come from the other side of the Tweed and starved like Texas temperance editors, returned rejoicing, and would have been cured just as effectually if a Devonshire dairyman had touched them up with his pitchfork. The true believers were mostly children of poverty who had come the long road afoot; and microbes that could have defied the shoulder hits of all the legitimate despots of Christendom had succumbed to a hunger-cure, intensified by liberal doses of active exercise.

Among the germ-diseases that have been relieved by fasting, the author of "The True Science of Living" also mentions malaria, eczema, gastric cancer, pneumonia and typhoid fever.

It is also a significant fact that the abstemious natives of the tropics are far less subject to the risk of blood-poison from severe wounds than the overfed children of civilization.

A germ-disease, as virulent as syphilis, and long considered too persistent for any but palliative methods of treatment (by mercury, etc.) was radically cured by the fasting cures, prescribed in the Arabian hospitals of Egypt, at the time of the French occupation. Avicena already alludes to the efficacy of that specific, which he seems to have employed with similar success against smallpox, and Dr. Robert Bartholow, a stickler for the faith in drugs, admits that "it is certainly an eminently rational expedient to relieve the organism of a virus by a continuous and gradual process of molecular destruction and a renewal of the anatomical elements. Such is the hunger-cure of syphilis, an Oriental method of treating that disease. Very satisfactory results have been attained by this means."—(Materia Medica and Therapeutics, pp. 31-32.)

The most mysterious of all disorders of the human organism, asthma, or respiratory paralysis, has been ascribed to November mists as often as to the debilitating influence of midsummer heat; but its proximate cause appears to have something to do with the accumulation of phlegm in the bronchial tubes, and its cure by abstinence, though slow, is far more permanent than the relief now and then obtained by the use of drugs. The villainous fumes of burning stramonium leaves, for instance, cause a convulsion of the respiratory apparatus which does break the asthma spell for the time being, but within half an hour after the patient has stopped panting and spitting the ominous torpor is apt to creep on again, and it has been noticed that with every repetition the doses of the distressing remedy has to be increased.

Denutrition, or total abstinence from solid food and all liquids but water, has no appreciable effect on respiratory paralysis for the first day or two, but before the end of the third day breathing becomes easier, the respirations, though weak, are freer, and before long become "deeper" and lung-filling enough to compensate the system for weeks of air-famine. One patient of my acquaintance had suffered such misery from suffocating fits that he felt as if the grip of a demon had been relaxed when his lungs began to work freer, and rather than forfeit his hard-won deliverance, hesitated to break his fast that day or the next. "I would rather drink my fill of air than of boarding- house coffee," he whispered, "and, as for hunger, I have really no time to notice the slight beginnings of that, I'm so busy feeling blest."

Fasters generally notice that the first two days of total abstinence are the worst, a sensation of general languor continues to increase, but by that time denutrition has begun to relieve all sorts of incidental affections, and the net result is a feeling of relief similar to that of a convalescent from a fever fit.

The effect of a fasting cure depends often upon its length, and upon no other point of an admittedly important problem the impressions of the general public are more contradictory and vague.

"You cannot expect a sick person to fast all day?" inquires Mrs. Hearsay, who would not hesitate to swallow sixteen different kinds of fashionable poisons.

In reply, Thomas Campanella states that frail nuns often sought relief from attacks of hysteria by fasting "seven times seventy hours," or twenty days and a half. Total abstinence for three weeks or more was not an uncommon prescription of Avicena, who was so averse to drastic remedies that he would sooner watch all night at the fever-bed of a patient than risk complications by the use of opiates. The great Arab was not an ascetic either. He detested unnecessary self-denial, so much so, indeed, that he advised his friends to miss no chance for fun on this side of the grave and set them convivial examples at the risk of incurring the wrath of Moslem zealots. Dr. Tanner, I believe, broke his thirty-nine days' fast by a midway glass of sweet lemonade, but Buddha Sakyammi, like his Galilean successor, fasted forty days even, just for the sake of clearing his brain.

The penance-worn saints of the early Christian Church thought nothing of retiring to the desert for a month or two, to fight down temptations and dine on the water of some dilapidated old cistern. To touch even millet-seed on such occasions was considered a breach of contract, forfeiting the merit of the enterprise, but at the end of the second month the gaunt world-renouncer had generally strength enough left to reach his convent unassisted and smash the solar plexus of a cell-brother who ventured to question the reality of his visions. Robert de Moleme, the founder of the Cistercian brotherhood, was overcome with grief on learning the death of a female friend, and like General Boulanger, resolved to follow her to the Land of Shades.

Being averse to direct suicide, he retired to the mountain-lodge of a relative, and abstained from food in the hope that one of his frequent fainting fits would fade into the sleep that knows no morning. But finding himself alive at the end of the seventieth day, he reconsidered his resolution and began to suspect a miraculous interposition of Providence. By resuming his meals, in half-ounce instalments, he contrived to recover from a condition of frightful emaciation, and in the supervision of an ever- increasing number of scattered monasteries, led an active life for the next fourteen years.

Trance-fasters, like Augusta Kerner of Ingolstadt, survived in a semi-conscious condition for nearly a quarter of a year, but it would be a mistake to suppose that staying powers of that kind are a prerogative of the sick. Miners in collieries, affording a sufficient supply of water, have been found alive after weeks of enforced abstinence from any more nutritious food than scraps of leather soaked in pit-water and masticated with desperate perseverance. Sailors, deprived of food and drink, have endured exposure to the glare of a tropical sun for a week or more. But the marvels of long-continued abstinence without loss of strength reach their maximum in the winter-sleep of several species of warm-blooded animals. Reptiles, with their small expenditure of vital energy, can easily survive dietetic deprivations, but bears and badgers, with an organization essentially analogous to that of the human species, and with a circulation of the blood active enough to maintain the temperature of their bodies more than a hundred degrees above that of the winter-storms, dispense with food for periods varying from three to five months, and at the termination of their ordeal emerge from their dens in the full possession of their physical and mental energies.*

* Karl Vogt in his "Curiosities of Instinct," mentions the case of a spaniel that had accidentally been locked up by

visitors to the attic of an old castle-ruin, and contrived to procure a few drops of water by gnawing the edges of a cleft in the slate-covered roof. His life had thus been saved by the accident of a few heavy rain-showers, but there was no chance for a crumb of food, no grain, leather, rats or mice, no vestige of living things with the exception of a few spiders under the rafters of the roof. The whole summer passed, and a part of autumn; but during the first week of October there was a picnic on the castle mountain, and a wandering party of sight-seers rescued the little prisoner that had been locked up about the middle of June. Its ribs could be counted as easily as in a skeleton, but it was still able to drag itself across the floor and lick the hands of its deliverers.

Chossat in his Recherches sur l'Inanition, states that the land tortoise of southern France can starve for a year without betraying a reduction of vital energy, and the Proteus anguinus, or serpent salamander, even for a year and a half, provided that the temperature of its cage be kept above the freezing point.

The black bear of northern Russia rolls itself up in scrap-heaps of leaves and moss, about the end of November, trusting to good luck to be left to the enjoyment of peaceful slumber till middle of March, but if disturbed before the end of February is wide awake in a minute and attacks the intruders with a fury expressed in a Slavonic phrase: equivalent to "savage as a waked winter bear." Badgers leave their burrows a little sooner, being often awakened by a spell of warm weather, a month before the vernal equinox, and after an absolute fast of ten weeks will trot for miles in search of roots and acorns that have perhaps to be scraped out of the half-frozen ground.

The little dormouse, in its winter-sleep of five months, suffers a loss of weight sometimes exceeding forty per cent., and exhibition fasters have survived a reduction of thirty per cent., without anything like a total collapse of vital vigor.

The first few meals after such a fast have to be served in doll-house saucers. Reckless gorging might forfeit all the advantages of a sanitary fast, and rations have to be raised from ounces to half pounds, with four-hour inter- vals—a precaution which Nature tries to enforce in a peculiar way of her own: After a fast of four days or more the teguments of the palate become so sensitive that mastication has to proceed with pauses.

The above quoted instances preclude the idea of a week's fast involving any life-endangering consequences. It would often relieve disorders which drugs can only complicate and give the patient a new lease of life, hope and vigor.

But for ordinary purposes even a two-days' intermission of surfeits would result in sanitary benefits apt to reform all but the most inveterate gluttons. No need of aggravating the sickness of dyspeptics by mentioning the "duty of self-denial," and evoke visions of spiritual advisers helping themselves to the assets of world-renouncing idiots; the mere change from physical misery and oppression to buoyancy and freedom would be sufficient to attain the approval of believers in happiness on this side of the grave.

During the last summer of Kitchener's campaign in the Soudan the Mahdists captured a British quartermaster, baggage and all, and, after harnessing him like a donkey, put him in a chain-gang of burden-carriers and loaded him up with a cargo of camping outfit and nigger babies. Pinching fetters, perspiration, and vermin completed the horrors of his predicament, and he was on the verge of suicide, when Captain Magruder's dragoons overtook his captors and celebrated his deliverance with a picnic at a spring. Washed, refreshed and dressed in cleanest linen, the freed man continued his journey rejoicing, but the contrast

43

of misery and comfort can hardly have surpassed that of a dyspeptic before and after a fasting-cure. The relief of his overburdened stomach has given Nature a chance to expurgate all sorts of encumbrances: accumulated ingesta, vitiated humors and sixteen different kinds of pinching, gnawing and excavating microbes. He feels as if a burden of rags and parasites had been removed from his shoulders; he can continue the pilgrimage of life without a handicap; his soul has been dressed in clean raiment.

And even from an epicuric point of view the revival of appetite would more than compensate a few days' abstinence. Food is relished to a degree that implies a pledge of its thorough assimilation. House-cleaning has prepared the storerooms for the reception of fresh supplies. The night's rest following the first appetite-sanctioned meal will not be disturbed by nightmares. Fasting, like exercise and refrigeration, makes repose sweet. The dull, unheeded, but ever-gnawing reproaches of the physical conscience have been silenced.

One great aid to the successful accomplishment of a fasting-cure is the rule to keep the mind as much as possible occupied, so as to prevent its brooding over the topic of alimentary deprivations; create some diversion by exciting pastimes or interest-absorbing work. Frederic Gerstaecker, in his "Chronicle of the Forty-niners," remarks that every nugget-bonanza lessened the temptations of intemperance. The miners were too busy to waste the golden chance on rum; they neglected the bar-room because they could find better excitement at the gravel-bar. They would hardly take time to eat their meals. The successful ones, especially, merely nibbled a crust and hurried back to work. After a cat-nap or two, they left their hammocks and opened the window-shutters as if they could hardly await the dawn of the morning. "Get up, boys, here's daylight at last," one of them would call out in the middle of the night; then, after scrutenizing the signs of the sky more closely: "Blame the luck, it's only the moon, after all."

It is, therefore, a good plan to reserve a specially diverting job of work for the term of a fasting-cure, but it should be remembered that severe physical efforts tend to complicate the demands upon the reserve energies of the organism. Tree-felling while fasting would be burning the candle of life at both ends. For similar reasons cold weather is apt to aggravate the ordeal of total abstinence. Winter is not the worst time for a fast, it may even be the best, to judge from the phenomena of hibernation; only it is well to recollect that in remedial effects two fasting- days, combined with exercise in a snow-storm, are equivalent to three fasting-days in midsummer.

The influence of habit tends to make abstinence easy—as easy almost as the dietetic restrictions which our gormandizing ancestors used to dignify by the name of fasting. Lenten fare, in the South-German sense of the word, came at last to imply only the shelving of flesh-pots, without excluding eggs, butter, cheese, oysters and fish, in any desired quantities. The greasy made dishes and eel-pies of the Bavarian refectories were perfect burlesques on the bona-fide fasts of the poor, and there is an anecdote about an Austrian granger who had attended a revival, and upon his return was seized with qualms of conscience at the sight of preparation for a feast of gravy dumplings. "Say, Jane, this is Good Friday," he muttered, "a dozen of those things is really too much for creatures who have souls to save. Make only ten, this time; but"—after some reflection—"you can make them a little larger than last week."

Yet with all their cart blanche of butter-pan dishes some slaves of habit contrived to get spiritual license for meat-rations on traveling-days, "on account of the extra fatigue and exposure to wind and weather."

45

But in the highlands of Algeria, in a climate almost as rigorous as that of the Alps, the soldiers of General Clausel were unable to procure meat, and after a few weeks' practice found, possibly to their own surprise, that they could get along very comfortably on dates, bread and cheese.

Eating only one meal a day becomes so much of a second nature, in a month or two, that habitues almost pity the slaves of custom who have to handicap their energies by forenoon surfeits. "Breakfast," if its etymology can be trusted, is a misnomer, where there has been no fast to speak of, and the idea of repletion before the day's work is done comes to appear as foolish as an invitation to a Saturday picnic at the beginning of the week. "Don't spoil your supper," whispers an inner monitor when the noonday pause awakens old-time associations, but after a little experience the contrast of present all-day buoyancy and former afternoon life-weariness is quite enough to nip temptations in the bud.

Abstinence from two meals has become natural enough to require no self-denial whatever, and in the course of time a fasting-cure expert can tackle the task of a two-days' term of total abstinence almost without a presentiment of discomfort. "A fishing-trip to-morrow evening will help me over the hill," he reflects, "and the next day I can eat with the assurance of digesting my supper to the last fraction of an ounce."

Even after a short fast the first full meal had better be preceded by a light lunch and a few hours' pause, to initiate the activity of the digestive organs, but the selection of a simple and perfectly digestible breakfast may modify the necessity of that precaution.

About the third week of Dr. Tanner's ordeal a Georgia sympathizer sent him an enormous watermelon that was wrapped up in newspapers and hidden in a corner of the room to mitigate the tantalizing effect of its presence. Visitors had almost forgotten its existence, but the moment his quarantine had been accomplished, the survivor got hold of that melon and proceeded to help himself with the energy of an Afro-American picnicker.

"Don't, sir, don't, screeched a Philadelphia dude, "you'll kill yourself in five minutes if you keep on like that."

"Hold on there, young man," said the old doctor, grabbing the meddler's arm, "I may be mistaken, but I believe I'm running this circus myself." But there was probably no mistake about it; a ripe watermelon is made up of about 97 per cent, of fluids to three of harmless solids, and the plucky faster's breakfast was almost as unobjectionable as a quart of sugar-water. The same quantum of hash might have killed him, and even the attempt to masticate a big piece of bread would have been baffled by the protest of the sensitive palate.

The question as to the requisite length of a remedial fast depends upon the previous habits of the experimenter. A glutton who has complicated the consequences of three daily surfeits by drastic drugs cannot hope to be restored to anything like a normal condition in less than a quarter of a year, devoted to three fasts of a week each, and with three-weeks' intervals of moderate eating and abundant outdoor exercise.

For an ordinary indigestion three days of total abstinence will generally suffice, and votaries of the one-meal plan can keep disease at bay with a two-days' fast at the end of every month. Provided that they abstain from greasy made-dishes and all abnormal stimulants that precaution will even save them the necessity of regulating the quantity of their meals after the plan of Louis Cornaro, who weighed out his daily rations with half-ounce scales. "Abstinence is easier than temperance," and a combination of the one-meal plan with an occasional fast is far more sensible, because more practicable, than everlasting self-denial.

A SEVEN-DAY FAST
CHAPTER V
AN EXPERIENCE OF ONE OF THE AUTHORS

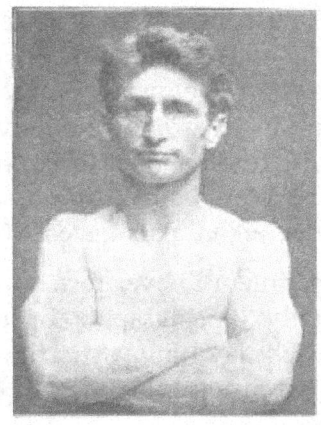

After Seven-day Fast

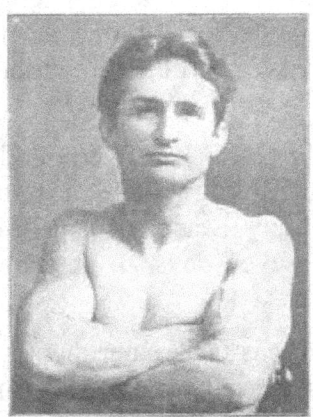

Normal Condition.

SHOWING HOW THE FACE WASTES DURING A FAST

The description of my fast of seven days, which appeared in "PHYSICAL CULTURE" some time ago, will probably be of interest to my readers.

During the last fifteen years I have frequently fasted as a cure for threatened illnesses that attack even the most careful in this age of civilized or rather uncivilized dietary.

I have been seriously threatened with pneumonia and numerous other ills of less importance which have quickly succumbed to this effective means of ridding the system of impurities. Though there are now some valuable works on this subject, when I first adopted these theories, they were based entirely on my own conclusion and instinct and the well-known fact that all animals fasted when ill.

Until this last experiment I never fasted over four days, and even then I usually ate an apple or a bite or two or something light each day, thus at no time previous to this last experiment did I fast absolutely.

I have frequently made comments on the value of fasting in "PHYSICAL CULTURE." and determined to test the effects of an absolute fast of one week on strength and weight. I did not take a particle of nourishment in any form, though drank freely of pure water.

The first day of the fast, I lost five pounds and the next day two pounds and the loss gradually decreased each day, and on the seventh day was but little over one pound. Altogether in the seven days, my total loss of weight was fifteen pounds.

My loss of weight was far greater than is usual when one is fasting. This was caused by the great amount of exercise that I took daily. In fact I lost about as much weight in this one week as one would ordinarily lose in two weeks if no exercise was taken.

Each day I walked about ten miles, and surprising as it may seem, I felt weaker the second day of the fast than at any time thereafter.

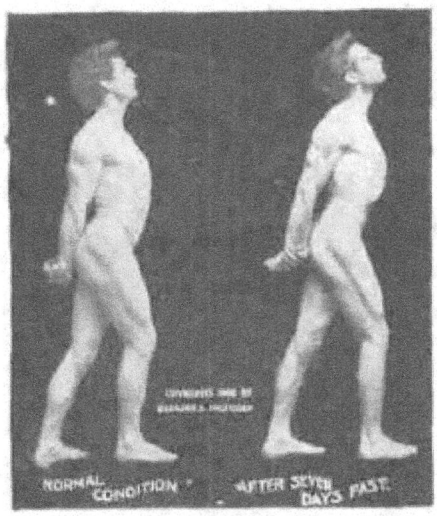

I always took my walk in the morning immediately on rising and usually felt weak at the start This was however entirely morbid, for after traveling one or two miles, it would entirely disappear and I could walk with a strong steady tread, and at the conclusion always felt equal to ten or twenty miles more.

Frequently when rising from a seat after a short rest 1 would feel quite dizzy for a few moments, but this would quickly pass away.

The first four days were the most uncomfortable. I did not seem especially hungry, but I was languid, except for a while after exercise at which times I always felt strong and energetic.

I attended to my daily duties during the entire fast with the same regularity as usual. My brain seemed especially clear, and mental work actually required less effort than when eating regularly.

At times difficulty was experienced in inducing sleep. The gnawing sensation in my stomach would not cease, though a plentiful supply of cool pure water seemed of great advantage, and was of valuable assistance in wooing slumber.

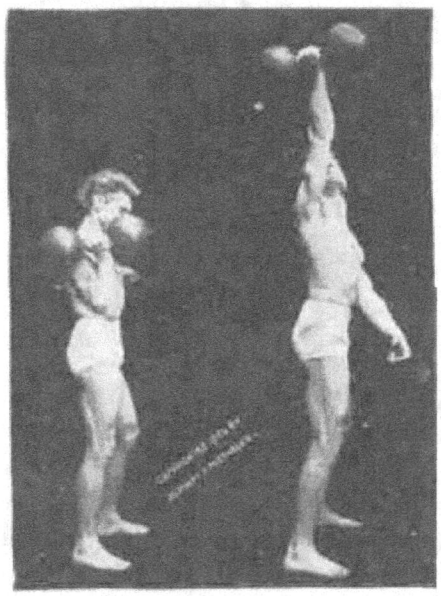

The sixth and seventh days of the fast were really by far the most comfortable. I felt that it would require but little effort to continue on for three or four weeks, but the object of the fast was accomplished and I was not at all anxious to continue it further.

The most important feature in lessening the effects of fasting is to keep the mind employed so one will not be continually referring to the desire for food.

The only time there was the slightest danger of my giving way to my appetite was on the fourth day. At this particular time I mention, there was nothing of importance for me to do and after conversing a short time with some friends, I went out with the distinct intention of patronizing the nearest restaurant.

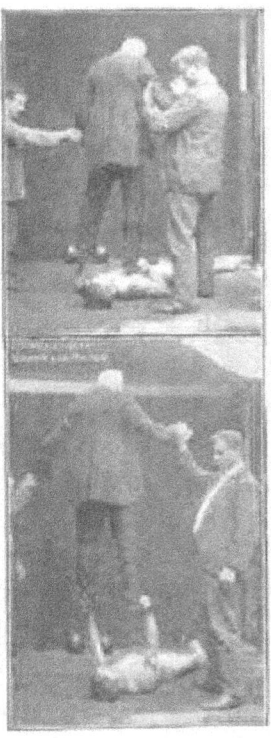

Raising 200-lb. man with strength of arms only, after seven-day fast.

After walking a short distance and giving the matter serious consideration, I determined not to break the fast and instead of the restaurant, I visited a gymnasium and spent thirty minutes in vigorous exercise, and in consequence felt much better, and all thoughts of giving up the fast were abandoned.

The comparison photographs show how the body wasted away during the fast. The face thinned especially and the eyes sunk considerably.

But the astounding fact in connection with the fast was the strength possessed on the seventh day. The average person imagines that he becomes weak even after missing a meal, and a fast of one day, is supposed to take away all strength. There was never greater error.

On the fourth day of the fast after testing my strength, I concluded to use a fifty pound dumb bell in illustrating my strength on the seventh day of the fast.

Well, the seventh day came at last, though I must confess the week seemed rather long. I visited the gymnasium after my walk with the intention of leaving instructions that the fifty-pound dumb bell be sent to the photographer's gallery. On arriving there, I felt so strong that I concluded to test my strength. I thought that may be I might be able to raise without difficulty a heavier bell than fifty pounds.

I raised the fifty-pound bell over my head a number of times without the slightest difficulty. It did not seem heavier than when at my usual weight. I tried the sixty-pound bell, then the seventy and eighty-five with similar results, and immediately left instructions to send the one-hundred-pound bell over to the gallery as I felt that my strength was equal to raising it.

I know full well that my readers will beamazed at these feats of strength performed after this long fast, and no one could be more amazed than I, for as stated before I was under the impression that to raise a fifty-pound bell over head with one hand after a fast of this character, would really be something worth boasting about, and I was astounded at my strength under the circumstances.

The hundred-pound dumb bell was sent to the gallery, and Sarony's employees who saw and photographed the feats will vouch for the statements made and the illustrations shown. I had to raise the hundred-pound dumb bell twice before a proper negative could be made of the feat.

The second feat of raising this 200-lb. man as shown in the photographs was not easy, as any one will discover on trial, and it would be well to remember that I never at any time in my athletic career believed in using heavy weights, and had not attempted to raise a hundred-pound dumb bell off the floor for at least two years previous to the performance of these feats.

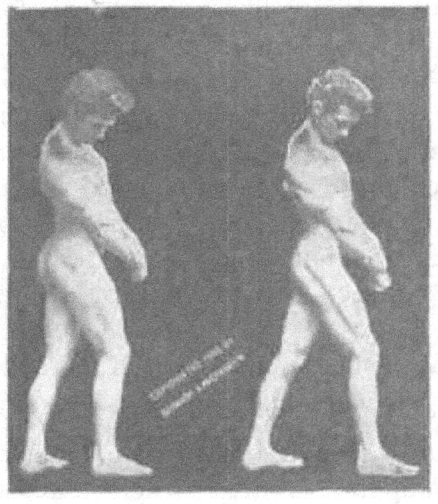

Normal Condition.   After Seven-day fast.

While in active practice in general athletic work a number of years ago, I could raise a hundred-pound bell eleven times at arms length over head with one arm, but at this time I occasionally handled these heavy weights. As I have taken no heavy exercise for a number of years, more than a slight effort would be required to raise this heavy dumb bell, even when my weight was at its usual standard.

A lesson is taught with unquestionable clearness by this experiment. The American people are actually eating themselves into their graves. Ninety-nine out of every hundred take from five to fifty years from the length of their lives by stuffing their stomachs. They eat, not to nourish the body, but merely for the pleasure of gourmandizing. The result is that from two to five times as much food passes through the alimentary canal than is necessary to maintain weight and strength, and mind and body are actually weakened by the strenuous efforts made by the system in endeavoring to rid itself of this excessive amount of food.

Any one can be benefited by a fast such as I describe here. Of course I would not advise one who has been eating three meals each day all during life to immediately attempt total abstinence from food for seven days, though such a fast under such conditions would be productive only of benefit provided it could be borne without too much of a mental strain and provided great care is used not to over-eat when normal dietary habits are resumed. In fact the greatest difficulty in connection with a fast of any duration is the tendency to over-eat after the fast. This error will often be productive of so much injury that all the beneficial results of a fast are practically nil.

After the fast I have described here I made the mistake myself of eating too heartily on two or three occasions and I am satisfied that much harm resulted thereby. On the second day after the fast I ate three hearty meals, when one hearty meal would have been sufficient. This was, as before mentioned, the first fast of this duration that I had ever gone through, and I was not prepared to meet conditions with which I was not familiar.

Unquestionably it would be better in experimenting with fasting to start by fasting one meal or say one day at a time. The result of this will give you confidence in its benefits, then you can gradually advance into a full-fledged convert. The principal result of value in such a conversion will be from that day forward absolute independence of all advisers, medical or otherwise, upon an ailment of any kind that attacks you. Fasting will be at once the principal part of your self-treatment, and forever thereafter your stomach will be free from the drug habit, and if you expect to retain the slightest respect for yourself you must first learn to respect your stomach.

II - HYDROTHERAPY
CHAPTER VI
PHYSIOLOGICAL DATA

Refrigeration is Nature's specific for the cure of germ-diseases, and the tardy recognition of that truth is certainly not justified by the lack of suggestive facts.

The first November frosts abate climatic fevers throughout the lowlands of the temperate zone. In the marshes of the Mississippi Valley agues that defy the remedies of the drug-store yield to the expurgative influence of a blizzard. North winds, reducing the temperature of the dog-days some forty degrees in as many minutes, bring a new lease of life to thousands of slum-tenants, to victims of chronic headaches, to infants exhausted by confinement in the sweltering atmosphere of city tenements. Refugees from cholera epidemics venture to return with the snowbirds.

And it is no accident that nine out of ten international wars ended with the victory of Northland tribes over their Southern neighbors. Egypt and Persia vanquished by Greeks, Greece by Romans, Rome by the barbarians of the Teutonic forests, South-German Austria by North-German Prussians, Southern Russia by the descendants of Ru- rik, Southern Italy by Savoy, South-Spanish Moors by North-Spanish Goths, Dixie by Yankeeland, South Mongol China by North-Mongol Japan. Highlanders, the world over, boast their superior vigor and longevity.

Physiology explains those facts and confirms the claim of the hydropathist Schrodt that refrigeration is one of the few natural tonics, stimulating the activity of the organic functions without the risk of deleterious aftereffects. A cold bath and a current of cold air accelerate the pulse and the process of respiration. The gasps resulting from a cold plunge-bath indicate the effort of Nature to restore the proper degree of animal warmth by setting the calorific apparatus to work under high pressure.

A dose of drastic drugs, e.g., alcohol in its concentrated forms, accomplish a similar result with almost equal promptness, the organism labors with feverish activity to rid itself of a life-endangering poison, and temporarily the whole system participates in the influence of the stimulant. But as soon as the problem of expurgation has been solved, a debilitating reaction sets in; the organism sinks under the exhausting aftereffects of the unnatural irritant, the mind is clouded by lingering poison-fumes, the depression of vital energy avenges itself by protracted languor, and the misery of mental gloom.

The benefits of the refrigeration tonic, on the other hand, are not modified by the risk of such penalties. The stimulating effect abides. And the first flush of that effect more than equals the bracing influence of the best drug-tonic. A cold bath renews the tension of nerve-vigor almost like refreshing sleep; its mental effect induces all the pleasant and none of the objectionable symptoms of intoxication.

Like fasting and exercise, hydrotherapy is a true remedy, relieving the ailments of the human organism without exacting a price that makes the cure a greater curse than the evil.

CHAPTER VII
THE COLD-WATER CURE

Hydrotherapy is one of the eldest offspring—perhaps the first-born—of natural hygiene. The desire to relieve the debilitating effects of summer heat by immersion and draughts of cold water is almost as instinctive as the craving for food. And it cannot have been long before the settlers of the higher latitudes noticed the fact that the health-impairing effects of indoor life could be counteracted by the same specific.

A cold bath restored the vigor of the Celtic hunter, emerging dazed from the turf-fumes of his cave-dwelling, and an old Austrian army-officer of my acquaintance was probably not the first toper who contrived to "sober up" at short notice by putting his head under the spout of a horse-pump. In midsummer repeated plunge-baths helped to obviate the risk of dietetic disorders, and as early as A.D. 550 free bathing facilities had come to be included among the principal desiderata of a civilized city. Athens, Corinth, Memphis, Agrigentum, and the great seaport towns of Western Asia had them; in Carthage they were maintained by a public tax and the voluntary contributions of numerous merchant-princes.

Imperial Rome became a Mecca of water-worshipers. Not less than six different aqueducts connected the city with the springs of wooded mountain-ranges—some of them twelve English miles from the corporation limits, and the Grand Therms of Caracalla atoned for all the demerits of the eccentric ruler; they formed a series of wall- enclosed artificial lakes, free to all, yet equipped with the conveniences of the most luxurious modern watering- place. The cold-water hall was large enough to accommodate the lovers of aquatic sports, and with its branch- tanks, in fact served the purpose of a swimming school.

Frequent baths were recognized as a main condition of physical welfare, and perhaps for that very reason were neglected by the bigots of an antinatural creed. The self-torturing monks gloried in filth, and Llorente, in his "History of the Inquisition," mentions numerous instances of converts from Mohammedanism incurring suspicion by continuing to practise the daily ablutions of their former faith. One ex-Morisco, a citizen of Cadiz, had a quarrel with a servant-girl, and soon after was arrested and jailed on a charge of apostasy. After being four times arraigned and as often scourged within an inch of his life, he was at last confronted with his accuser. In her thirst for revenge, the slandermonging slut had denounced him as a backslider and supported her insinuations with the assertion that her former employer was in the habit of locking himself up and taking a bath thrice a week. By sacrificing half his fortune and summoning a dozen medical witnesses, the defendant escaped the stake on a plea of physical necessity; his duties as manager of a woolen mill, he proved, obliged him to avoid cutaneous troubles by extra sanitary precautions, which he otherwise abhorred as practices of benighted misbelievers.

All over the Mediterranean coastlands free public baths were in ruins; but the belief in the concomitance of godliness and dirt does not seem to have been limited to Southern Europe. "Bathing, being pleasant as well as wholesome," says Henry Buckle, in his description of Scotch kirk-despotism," was considered a particularly grievous offense; and no man could be allowed to swim on Sunday. It was, in fact, doubtful whether swimming was lawful for a Christian at any time, even on week days, and it was certain that God had on one occasion shown his disapproval by taking away the life of a boy while he was indulging in that carnal practice." ("History of Civilization," Vol. II., p. 312.)

" As bathing was a heathenish custom, all public baths were to be destroyed" (by order of the Inquisition) "and even all larger baths in private houses." (Ibid., Vol. II., p. 44.)

That millennium of insanity left its traces in the still far-spread mistrust of out natural instincts, and not before the middle of the eighteenth century a revival of common sense led to the re-establishment of free public baths in several cities of Holland and Southern Europe. Watering-places became fashionable, but the choice of the public favored warm springs, till Squire Priessnitz, a self-educated farmer of Graefenberg, Silesia, called attention to the remedial efficacy of cold-water prescriptions. In his private sanitarium—a mere annex, at first, of a homely farm-house—he used shower-baths, sponge-baths, sitz-baths, and internal doses of pure water from a cold mountain spring, and proved that for the treatment of debilitating disorders his prescriptions made drugs superfluous.

The theories of the water doctor, as his neighbors called him, were founded on personal experience. Soon after taking charge of a small farm he had been all but killed in a runaway accident. His survival seemed doubtful, and when he left the hospital of a neighboring city he "was a mere bundle of disabilities," stiff-jointed, half lame, and troubled with all sorts of pains and disorders. A swollen foot having been greatly benefited by immersion in cold water, the convalescent tried the effect of an occasional sitz-bath, then of daily all-over sponge-baths, and before the end of the second year had got rid of all his ailments. As far as he could remember, he had, indeed, never felt better in his life, except in early boyhood when a relative now and then took him out to a berry-picking camp in the highlands, and the little lad "wondered if the dwellers in paradise could have been much happier."

In his subsequent school-years he used to take long rambles all by himself, feeling more at home in the mountain cliffs than in the tobacco-clouded village tavern—evidently a child of Nature, with the very instincts that would lead him to abandon drug-traditions for a new gospel of hygiene.

He was no learned man, in the college sense of the word, but had read a good deal and thought more, and his arguments had the force born of intense conviction. Besides, his own experience was an argumentum ad hominem, and one by one his afflicted neighbors tried the inexpensive prescriptions of the water-doctor. Reformed topers felt their shattered nerves braced as no drugs, no ointments and strengthening diet had braced them before. Rickety youngsters improved till they could join in the sports of their contemporaries and often beat them at their own game. Invalids with one foot in the grave regained their vantage ground on the upper tablelands of health, and one

old soldier became so enthusiastic a champion of the new sanitary creed that his savage denunciations of drug-mongers more than once got him into serious trouble.

Squire Priessnitz himself never indulged in invectives, and kept his temper even when the neighboring physicians got him indicted for kur pfuscherie—the unauthorized practise of medicine; "mal-practice" being a term they could not apply to his case, as there were no plaintiffs and it could not be proved that anybody had ever been the worse for a cold-water cure. The sympathy of the public was emphatically on the side of the defendant, who relied on his native eloquence and asked the court if it was fair to force an indictment for the practise of medicine against a man who had never encouraged the belief in the efficacy of medicinal prescriptions or dispensed a grain of drugs in his life. "Bathing," he argued, "is a mere sanitary habit, and you might as well arrest me for advising my neighbors to take more outdoor exercise or try a change of diet."

Those neighbors became a trifle too demonstrative in their applause, and the court warned all concerned to "be more careful hereafter," but, on the whole, thought it best to discharge the prisoner.

The kreis physicus (chief health officer of the district) threatened to appeal the case, but at the urgent advice of a legal friend, concluded to desist.

As a net result of the prosecution, Squire Priessnitz gained so many new patrons that he had to enlarge his sanitarium, and the next year could add a new branch for female patients. As usual in such cases, the charm of novelty attracted additional customers from ever-increasing distances, and two years before his death the now old "water doctor" could boast of having eight patients from France and two from the Netherlands. Women, strange to say, came to outnumber the male visitors, though probably only after Priessnitz had modified his rather heroic routine of prescriptions in favor of hysterical patients.

We should add a few words about the fierce controversy which a few years after Priessnitz's death was excited by the attempt to suppress the "water-cures" which in the meantime had sprung up all over Western Europe. The indignation of the hydropaths now and then rose to a pitch of fury, but their grievance was really worse than the proverbial provocation of saints. In Las Casas' "History of the West Indian Colonies" an eyewitness describes the numerous victims of Spanish despotism, as worn-out fugitives who could be seen perishing in way-side ditches, and faintly crying "Hunger, hunger!"

Even thus the lovers of truth had been persecuted and starved for a long series of centuries. Opponents of the autocrat swindle were slain as rebels. Dissenters from the insanities of the ghost-swindle were burned as heretics. Protests against the delusions of the drug-swindle were silenced by the bullies of the government quack-ring. For the coalition of shams had developed a union of state and drug-stores as oppressive and jealous as the union of State and Church, though the practise of medicine at last almost deserved the stigma of licensed murder.

"Die oft mit ihren hoellischen Latwergen In diesen Thaelern, diesen Bergen, Weit schlimmer als die Pest gehaust," says Goethe in the Prologue of "Faust"—"with their hellish nostrums they raged worse than the very pestilence."

After a thousand years' reign of Bruno's "Bestia trionfante," the blatant beast of Imposture—truth, for the first time, had got in a word edgeways; one small standard of fact and naturalism had been raised and successfully defended against the swashbucklers of shams. Can we wonder that all friends of reform rushed to its support and repelled aggression as the refugees of an island, rising above the waves of a universal deluge, would repulse an attack of sea-monsters?

Truth, for once, prevailed. Hydrotherapy contrived to hold its own against all comers, and health-seekers could rejoice in the certainty of having found a true remedy for a number of disorders which thus far had been only complicated and aggravated by conventional prescriptions.

No observer, unbiased by hearsay prejudices, could doubt that Priessnitz had discovered a reliable specific for the cure of dyspepsia and nervous debility, for sick headaches, insomnia, and the disorders resulting from overheating and protracted indoor life.

It is true of the hydrotherapists of the nineteenth century have in several respects modified the methods of the Silesian doctor; but it is also certain that the objections against the main principles of the system have been successfully refuted. There is no danger in three-minute immersions, followed by an energetic use of the towel, and no harm can result from reducing the temperature of the bath to 50° Fahrenheit—least of all in midsummer. The supposed peril of plunge-baths or draughts of cold water "in the heat," is one of the silliest bugbears of sanitary superstition. Shall we be asked to believe that the most natural of all beverages could become health-endangering when the voice of instinct clamors most urgently for refrigeration? The preposterous absurdity of the idea is rebuked by the example of our instinct-guided fellow-creatures who in warm weather, and after hours of strenuous exercise, drink their fill of cold spring-water, without the slightest hesitation and without any appreciable injurious consequences. Children, admonished not to touch cold water till they are cooled off, might as well be warned against falling asleep when they are tired.

And it is the same with cold baths. Professor Tyndale, in his "Hours of Recreation in the Alps," notices the astonishment of his Swiss guides who saw him plunge into the deep pool of a mountain torrent, after climbing uphill all afternoon in the glare of an August sun. "Their objections," he observes, "seemed to be founded on the difference in the temperature of the sun-heated atmosphere and that of the shaded brook, but that very contrast guaranteed the safety of the venture. In cold weather, when the organism is already suffering from the difficulty of maintaining its inner warmth at the proper medium, a cold bath might have overtaxed the vital staying powers; in midsummer there is no such risk." And training will even reduce the peril of winter baths to a safe minimum. Nay, the stimulating effect of the reflux of animal warmth (assisted by friction and brisk exercise) is perhaps most noticeable in moderately cold weather; and there are scores of habitues who take plunge-baths in ice-covered rivers to enjoy the subsequent glow of health, and maintain that the practise is the most reliable of all safeguards against the risk of "taking cold."

Cold baths incidentally also serve the purpose of a cosmetic. "I would undertake to identify hydropa- thists of the heroic school by their complexions," says Professor Carl Vogt; "and I have known octogenarians who had preserved the bloom of youth by the persistent use of ice-water."

Bathing, followed by the use of a coarse towel, stimulates the action of the skin to a degree that enables it to facilitate the work of the respiratory organs. Our pores have aptly been called supplementary lungs, and all sorts of impurities are secreted by cutaneous exhalations, as well as by the breathing process.

Water of almost any temperature compatible with comfort would subserve that special end, but only cold water tends to expurgate microbes. Cold sponge-baths have often sufficed to nip an attack of climatic fevers in the bud; and Dr. Sydenham mentions the case of three smallpox patients who were capsized on the way to an island pest- house, and in spite of (almost certainly because of) their involuntary ice-water bath, recovered with a facility unprecedented in the records of the lazaretto.

Two baths a day, one early in the morning, the other just before supper, is the usual routine of our hydropathic health-resorts, which, besides, prescribe liberal internal doses of cold spring-water. Common sense is bidding fair to prevail against prejudice in regard to the use of cooling beverages in febrile diseases, the world over, and one of our largest American sanitariums (managed mainly on an eclectic plan of reform) now offers its nurses premiums for persuading sufferers from various disorders to drink a maximum quantity of pure cold water.

The stronghold of the drug-delusion, indeed, is getting breached from all sides, but the leaders of the most nu- merous storming party must plead guilty to the charge of having recruited their ranks by manifold concessions to

67

popular errors. Hydrotherapy has thus far not attained the front rank of progress by a numerical test of success, but its victories can certainly claim prestige as triumphs of uncompromising truth.

CHAPTER VIII
AIR BATHS

In the cure of diseases by refrigeration, cold air is the readiest substitute for cold water. In the higher latitudes Nature supplies the remedy free of cost for six months of each year, and intermittently hundreds of times even in midsummer and at the threshold of the tropics, for the reduction of temperature in the early morning hours generally suffices to restore the functional vigor of the jaded organism.

The remedial effect of cold air equals that of cold water; air-cures, indeed, offer the advantage of superior facility of application for the cure of respiratory disorders. Expurgative currents of cold air can be made to reach the tissue of the lungs, and the significance of that circumstance is commensurate with the prevalence of a delusion more mischievous than the drug-superstition, vis.: the current theories concerning the cause of catarrh and consumption.

"Consumption," says an advocate of medical reform, "is a house-disease, and the plan of confining its victim in overheated, ill-ventilated sickrooms favors the development of its germs to a degree which the remedial powers of Nature strive in vain to counteract. . . . Not drugs or warmth, but cold, pure air is Nature's specific for the cure of consumption and ' colds.'"

That "colds," or catarrhal affections, are so very common— so much, indeed, as to be considerably more frequent than all other diseases taken together—is mainly due to the fact that the cause of no other disorder of the human organism is so generally misunderstood. Few persons have recognized the origin of yellow fever; about the primary cause of asthma we are yet all in the dark; but in regard to "colds" alone the prevailing misconception of the truth has reached the degree of mistaking the cause for a cure, and the most effective cure for the cause of the disease. If we inquire after that cause, ninety-nine patients out of a hundred, and at least nine out of ten physicians, would answer: "Cold weather," "raw March winds," or "cold draughts"—in other words, outdoor air of a low temperature. If we inquire after the best cure, the answer would be, "Warmth and protection against cold draughts"—i. e., warm, stagnant, indoor air.

And yet it can be proved with as absolute certainly as any physiological fact admits of being proved, that warm, vitiated indoor air is the cause, and cold outdoor air the best cure of lung-disorders. Many people "catch cold" every month in the year, and often two or three times a month. Very few get off with less than three colds a year; so that an annual average of five catarrhs would probably be an under-estimate. For the United States alone that would give us a yearly aggregate of three hundred and fifty-five million "colds."

That such facilities for investigation have failed to correct the errors of our exegetical theory is surely a striking proof how exclusively our dealings with disease have been limited to the endeavor of suppressing the symptoms, instead of ascertaining and removing the cause. For, as a test of our unbiased faculty of observation, the degree of that failure would lead to rather unpronounceable conclusions. What should we think of the scientific acumen of a traveler who, after a careful examination of the available evidence, should persist in maintaining that mosquitoes are engendered by frost and exterminated by sunshine?

Yet, if his attention had been chiefly devoted to the comparative study of mosquito ointments and mosquito bars, he might, for the rest, have been misled by such circumstances as the fact that gnats abound near the icy shores of Hudson Bay and are rarely seen on the sunny prairies of Southern Texas.

In all the civilized countries of the colder latitudes, catarrhs are frequent in winter and early spring, and less frequent in midsummer: hence, the inference that catarrhs are caused by cold weather and can be cured by warm air.

Yet of the two fallacies, the mosquito theory would, on the whole, be the less preposterous mis' take, for it is true that long droughts, by parching out the swamps, may sometimes reduce the mosquito plague; but no kind of warm weather will mitigate a catarrh, while the patient persists in doing what thousands never cease to do the year round, namely, to expose their lungs, night after night, to the vitiated, sickening atmosphere of an unventilated bedroom. "Colds" are, indeed, less frequent in midwinter than at the beginning of spring. Frost is such a powerful disinfectant that in very cold nights the lung-poisoning atmosphere of few houses can resist its purifying influence; in spite of padded doors, in spite of "weather-strips" and double windows, it reduces the indoor temperature enough to paralyze the floating disease-germs.

The penetrative force of a polar night-frost exercises that function with such resistless vigor that it defies the preventive measures of human skill; and all Arctic travelers agree that among the natives of Iceland, Greenland, and Labrador pulmonary diseases are actually unknown.

Protracted cold weather thus prevents epidemic catarrh; but during the first thaw Nature succumbs to art; smouldering stove fires add their fumes to the effluvia of the dormitory; tight-fitting doors and windows exclude the means of salvation; superstition triumphs, the lung-poison operates, and the next morning a suffering, coughing, and red-nosed family discuss the cause of their affliction. "Taken cold"— that much they premise, without a debate. But where and when? Last evening, probably, when the warm south wind tempted them to open the window for a moment. Or, "when those visitors kept chatting on the porch and a drop of water from the thawing roof fell on my neck." Or else, the boys caught it by playing in the garden and not changing their stockings when they came home. Resolved, that a person cannot be too careful as long as there is any snow on the ground. But even that explanation fails in spring, and when the incubatory influence of the first moist heat is brought to bear on the catarrh-germs of a large city, a whole district-school is often turned into a snuffling congress. The latter part of March is the season of epidemic catarrhs, and the evil is ascribed to "dampness," when the cold-theory becomes at last too evidently preposterous.

To an unprejudiced observer that theory, though, is equally untenable in the coldest months of the year. No man can freeze himself into a catarrh. Out-of-doors we cannot "catch cold."

"I have, upon the approach of cold weather, removed my undergarments," says Dr. Charles Page, "and have then attended to my outdoor affairs, minus the overcoat habitually worn; I have slept in winter in a current blowing directly about my head and shoulders; upon going to bed, I have sat in a strong current, entirely nude, for a quarter of an hour, on a very damp, cold night, in the fall of the year. These and similar experiments I have made repeatedly, and have never been able to catch cold. I became cold, sometimes quite cold, and became warm again, that is all. ("Natural Cure," p. 40.)

There are many ways, less often sought than found, for "becoming quite cold and warm again," but an experimenter, trying to contract a catarrh in that manner, would soon give it up as a futile enterprise; after two or three attempts he would find the attainment of his purpose more hopeless than before; he would find that instead of impairing, he had improved the functional vigor of his breathing-apparatus. Cold is a tonic that invigorates the respiratory organs when all other stimulants fail.

As soon as oppression of the chest, obstruction of the nasal ducts, and unusual lassitude indicate that a "cold has been taken"—in other words, that an air-poison has fastened upon the bronchi—its influence should at once be counteracted by the purest and coldest air available, and the patient should not stop to weigh the costs of a day's furlough against the danger of a chronic catarrh. In case imperative duties should interfere, the enemy must be met after dark, by devoting the first half of the night to an outdoor campaign and the second half to an encampment before a wide-open window.

There is no doubt that the proximate cause of a catarrh consists in the action of some microscopic parasite that develops its germs while the resistive power of the respiratory organs is diminished by the influence of impure air. Cold air arrests that development by direct paralysis; i.e., by lethargizing and eventually destroying the vitality of the disease-germs. Towards the end of the year a damp, sultry day—the catarrh-weather par excellence—is some-times followed by a sudden frost, and at such times I have often found that a six-hours' inhalation of pure, cold night-air will free the obstructed air-passages so effectually that on the following morning hardly a slight huskiness of the voice remains to suggest the narrowness of the escape from a two-weeks' respiratory misery.

It would be a mistake to suppose that "colds" can be propagated only by direct transmission, or the breathing of recently vitiated air. Catarrh germs, floating in the atmosphere of an ill-ventilated bedroom, may preserve their vitality for weeks after the house has been abandoned, and the next renter should not move in till the whole building has been subjected to an air-bath, and till wide-open windows and a through-draught of several days has re-moved every trace of a "musty" smell.

About the comparative advantages of dry and moist ("marine") climates opinions are divided, with a preponder-ance of argument in favor of the former, but so much is certain that for the cure of lung-complaints a low tempera-ture, with or without an excess of atmospheric moisture, is preferable to the perennial heat of the tropics. "I shall not attempt to explain," says Benjamin Franklin, "why damp clothes occasion colds, rather than wet ones, because I doubt the fact; I believe that neither the one nor the other contributes to this effect, and that the causes of catarrhs are totally independent of wet, and even of cold." ("Miscellaneous Works," p. 216.)

Nor can drugs compensate the lack of Nature's specific. In the language of our instincts every feeling of discomfort suggests its own remedy. If the proximity of a glowing stove begins to roast your shins, the alarmed nerves cry out—not for patent ointments, not for anti-caustic liniments and "pain-killers," but for a lower temperature Nothing else will permanently appease them. Millions of prisoners, school-children and factory-slaves, pine for lung-food as a starving man yearns for bread, and that hunger cannot be stilled with cough-pills, but only with fresh air.

Pure cold air is also a sovereign remedy for digestive disorders. The assimilative capacity of the human organism increases with the distance from the equator. An Esquimaux can digest a quantum of food that would crapulate three Hottentots and six Hindus. Camping in the open air whets the appetite even without the aid of active exercise. A bracing temperature exacts a sort of automatic exercise: It accelerates the circulation, it promotes the oxidation of the blood, and stimulates the whole respiratory process. The generation of animal caloric has to be increased to balance the depression of the external temperature. Hence the invigorating effect of mountain air and of sea- voyages. The first dose of the tonic can be applied in-doors by gymnastics in the ancient sense of the word that implies exercise in a state of nudity ("gymnos," in Greek, meaning simply "naked")—a few minutes' pause between undress and bedtime.

People who have got rid of the night-air superstition can almost defy dyspepsia by sleeping in a cross-draught, or in cold weather at least near a half-open window. Cold, fresh air is an invaluable aid to the assimilation of non-nitrogenous articles of food (fat meat, butter, etc.). Stifling bedrooms neutralize the effects of outdoor exercise. Winter is, therefore, on the whole the most propitious time for beginning a dyspepsia cure. In summer a highland sanitarium is the best place to start with; or, for coast-dwellers, a breezy sea-shore.

The efficacy of an air-bath as a cure of insomnia is suggested by the hypnotic influence of refrigeration. At least a dozen different species of our North American mammals get drowsy enough in cold weather to go to sleep about the end of November and postpone their awakening till spring. We sleep sounder in winter than at any other time of the year, and Dr. Franklin, who, like Bacon and Goethe, had the gift of anticipative intuitions, recommends air sitz-baths as an excellent substitutes for opiates. "In summer-nights, when I court sleep in vain," he says, "I often get up and sit at the open window or at the foot of my bed, stark-naked for a quarter of an hour. That simple expedient removes the difficulty (whatever its cause), and upon returning to bed I can generally rely upon getting two or three hours of most refreshing sleep."

It can, however, do no harm to combine an air-bath with a few minutes of indoor exercise. Perfect freedom of motion is, indeed, incompatible with the restraint of artificial teguments, and the effect of Dr. Franklin's prescription could generally be improved by gymnastics tending to stimulate the action of the respiratory organs. During sleep the blood is only imperfectly oxidized, and an accumulated deficiency of that sort (indicated by choking fits) is one of the most common causes of interrupted slumber.

The solaria, or sunbath-rooms of the ancients, probably served a similar purpose. Stoves and chimney fires— though not unknown—were rare in Athens, and in Rome were considered a prerogative of wealth; the great plurality, even of well-to-do citizens, survived the winter under a load of cumbersome garments, and now and then retired to a solarium to give their skins a chance for direct contact with the circulation-stimulating atmosphere.

CHAPTER IX
CLIMATIC SANITARIA

Wet feet, especially feet wetted by a walk in the chill dew of a meadow, ranked with the chief sanitary bugbears of our forefathers, and that a bugbear of that sort should now be ridden as a fashionable hobby is certainly an encouraging sign of the times. It proves at all events that hygienic prejudices are not unconquerable, but the mass-pilgrimages to the meadows of Woerishofen in Southern Germany make it evident that—well, that not all of our fellow-Caucasians have a right to poke fun at Charley Lambs' house-burning Chinamen. A citizen of Qwang-Soo, according to the most immortal essay of the gentle "Eliah," once found the remains of a cremated pig in the ruins of a burnt dwelling, and, ecstasized by a taste of the crust, hastened to spread the tidings of great joy. Pork, thus far, had always been eaten raw, and opinions differed as to the propriety of improving its flavor by a deviation from a time-honored custom. The cremation party at last prevailed, and even secured the sanction of legislators, but every time they felt a hankering after roast spare-ribs they thought it necessary to set a house afire.

Yet the price of an old Chinese farmstead cabin can hardly have exceeded that of an American ticket to Woerishofen, where the presiding priest of the new temple of health compels his converts to perform barefoot gallop- ades in a wet clover-field. No doubt a good many of them do get their money's worth in improved health, but the physiological value of Father Kneipp's prescription is simply that of a refrigeration cure, and every one of his forty-odd thousands of yearly visitors—some of them from distant Canada—would have derived exactly the same amount of benefit from a sponge-bath in the woodshed of his native ranch. The hindfoot plan of the Woerishofen prophet is, in fact, nothing but localized hydrotherapy, out and out less efficacious that the system of Squire Priessnitz, and efficacious at all only by virtue of long-continued repetitions. Special virtues of dew-moisture? Of South-German varieties of clover? Believe it, if you can, but stop smiling at Qwang-Soo pork procedures.

All there is of sense in the semi-mystic circulars of the clover-patch ^sculapius is founded on the fact that the early morning may be a specially propitious time for hydropathic transactions; the patients' lungs get the benefit of the cool morning air while his body is revelling in the pond of Siloam, or his feet in the parsonage pasture.

And since cool mornings are rare in the summer season of our lowlands, the "mountain cure" has a legitimate claim to the attention of health-seekers, especially where highlands have preserved their wealth of air-filtering forests. Carbonic acid, the lung-poisoning residium of respiration and combustion, is heavier than the atmospheric air, and accumulates in low places—in wells, in cellars, in deep, narrow valleys, etc.—and often mingles with the malarious exhalations of low, swampy plains. On very high mountains, on the other hand, the air becomes too rarefied to be breathed with impunity. It causes a spasmodic acceleration of the respiratory process, and is, therefore, especially distressing to diseased (wasted) lungs, whose functions are already abnormally quickened, and cannot be further stimulated without overstraining their mechanism.

In the temperate zone the purest and at the same time most respirable air is found at an elevation of about four thousand feet above the level of the sea—an altitude corresponding to the midway terraces of the European Alps, and the average summit-regions of our Southern Alleghanies. The broad tablelands of the Cumberland Range are several hundred feet above the dust and mosquito level.

Between the thirty-fourth and thirty-sixth degrees of north latitude the elevated plateaux have the further advantage of a climate that equalizes the contrasts of the seasons: it mitigates the summer more than it aggravates the winter.

Southerly winds predominate, and melt the snow with the same breezes that cool the midsummer weeks, for in the dog-days the Mexican tablelands are considerably cooler than our Northern prairie States.

Night frosts, it is true, occur a month earlier in the lowlands, but mark the beginning of the season when a sojourn in a mountain camp attains its maximum of sanitary benefit. How absurdly the risk of a bivouac in the snow has been overrated, may be inferred from the fact that the rumor of several miraculous cures a few years ago attracted hundreds of consumptives to winter-camps in the upper Adirondacks, in a climate quite as rigorous as that of Western Canada. They lived in tents, most of them, and passed the days hunting and snow-shoveling, and the nights comfortably enough under twenty woolen blankets, if a dozen were not sufficient, and all faithfully following Dr. Dio Lewis' plan of giving the ice-cold and ice-pure highland air a chance to expurgate their microbe-ridden lungs. Invalids who would have coughed away their lives in a tropical swamp-resort recovered in these cloud-land camps—not men only but women and feeble children. It has, indeed, often been observed that the moral effect of protracted confinement in a hospital is not favorable to the chances of recovery, and, moreover, a private establishment lessens the danger of contagion. And in the highlands of North Carolina, Tennessee, and Northern Georgia land and labor are so cheap that even people of moderate means can build a sanitarium of their own.

A log house can be made as airy as any tent, and is out and out more comfortable. A rough-hewed porch-roof, projecting like the veranda of a Swiss chalet, will keep the cabin both dry and airy, square holes in the center of each wall can serve as windows in fine weather, and during a storm can be kept shut with a sliding board. Between May and November the winds of the Southern Alleghanies come from the south or southwest, and in order to get the full benefit of the pure air, the house should face the plain from one of the thousand promontories that rise above the terrace-land of the "Piedmont country." Have the door on the south side and keep it wide open all night, as well as the windows or louvres in the opposite wall. If the windows do not reach to the ground, spread your bedclothes upon a hurdle bedstead, rather than on the floor, in order to enjoy the full current of the night-breeze.

Night and day one can thus breathe mountain airs that have not been tainted by the touch of earthly things since they left the pine forests of the Mexican Sierras. Every inspiration is a draught from the fountain-head of the atmospheric stream.

There is no need of living on oiled sardines where the brooks are full of speckled trout. Those who must break the commandment of Brahma (and the highland air confers certain immunities) may devour their humble relatives in the form of wild turkeys, quails, and 'possums, but the products of the vegetable kingdom are cheap and diversified enough to make up a tolerable menu. Sweet potatoes at 12 cents a peck, string beans 15, green peas 25, strawberries 10 cents a quart.

Whortleberries "huckleberries") are sold at 10 cents a gallon, but the pleasure of picking them is worth a great deal more. The lamest and weakest can join in that sport, for the shrub attains a height of three feet, and thus saves one the trouble of stooping, to conquer health by that utilitarian method.

Whenever the weather becomes too warm to guarantee the benefit of the enterprise on the main point, air baths should be supplemented by plunge baths in one of the pools of the never-failing mountain brooks. In the great forest-preserves of our East American highlands every glen has a rivulet of its own, born in the Land of the Sky, and preserving the temperature of its headwaters in the shade of spruce-pines, laurel-thickets, and overhanging rocks. Tellico River, with its fountain in the summit regions of the Unakas, at the border of Tennessee and North Carolina, is still as cold as spring-water where it issues from the foothills, fifteen miles further west, and there are fine bathing pools on the very plateaux, especially those of the Cumberland Range, which at several points north of Chattanooga attains a width of ten miles, with midway dells and hillocks.

Nor is there any lack of opportunities for trying Professor Tyndall's combination of cooling baths with blood-warming exercise. The choice between the various chances for entertaining work is the only difficulty, for Nature has provided them in embarrassing profusion. Expert bee-hunters can find three or four hive trees in a single clay. The chestnut forests of the upper ridges are full of squirrels, and with a dog, a sack, and a good axe it is not difficult to catch one alive and turn it over to the quartermaster of the pet department. Climbing trees is an exercise that brings in action nearly every muscle of the human body, and, like the mal de monte, the shudder that seizes the traveler at the brink of Alpine precipices, the dizziness that takes away the breath returns it with interest and is a mechanical asthma-cure.

Entomologists may combine the gratification of their mania with useful exercise by rolling logs in quest of stag- horn beetles. Log-rolling and tumbling rocks from the tops of projecting cliffs is the spice of life in the engineering enterprises which a camp full of male North Americans are sure to set afoot—such as enlarging the entrance of a cave, constructing a graded trail to the next spring, to the next wagon-road, or to a favorite lookout point.

Enterprises of that sort involve a good deal of grubbing and chopping, but a suit of Turner Khaki makes work pleasant. The despotism of fashion is not recognized in mountain camps. A pair of linen trousers, a hunting shirt, and loose necktie suffice for a hygienic summer-dress. In the afternoon remove the necktie and roll up the sleeves. It can do no harm to imbibe fresh air by all available means and let the cutaneous lungs share in the luxury. Nor is there any excuse for the widespread fallacy that it is dangerous, even in the most sultry nights, to remove the bed-blankets. Kick them into the farthest corner if they become too warm, and sleep in your shirt and drawers, or under a linen bed-sheet. Half-naked lazzaroni sleep the year round on the stone terrace of the Museo Borbonico, and outlive the asthmatic burghers in their sweat-box dormitories.

The body effects part of its breathing through the pores. Painting a man all over with yellow ochre and copal varnish would kill him as surely as hanging him by the neck. The confined air between the sleeper's body and a stratum of heavy blankets gets gradually surcharged with carbonic acid—in warm weather even to the verge of the saturation-point. The perspiration is thus forced back upon the body; and the lungs—perhaps already weakened by disease—have to do double work.

"Hier bin ich Mensch, hier darf ich's sein." says Goethe's "Faust," in his mountain retreat, and a prejudice- defying friend of mine makes no scruple of arising from the pallet of his summer-camps and roaming the moonlit woods in the costume of Adam, drinking in oxygen through every pore, and wondering if the longevity of the ancients had not something to do with the fact that they could enjoy air-baths of that sort all summer, and not in moonlight only.

CHAPTER X

VENTILATION

A traveling revivalist displays charts of the Eastern continents to illustrate the vast area of territories still in need of missionary labors. The extent of the field for sanitary reform might be realized by any observer strolling the streets of a large city in the twilight of a summer morning. In the tropics—even on the cool tablelands of Northern Mexico, he would see thousands of sleepers encamped upon the texadas, or flat roofs of their dwelling-houses; but in the United States, in Great Britain, France, Germany and Austria he would see 999 of a 1000 windows tightly closed, even in a temperature making indoor confinement positive torture.

"Night air? What are you afraid of?" asked Miss Florence Nightingale in her reports from the Crimean hospitals; "do you suppose God's free air is made deadly by the temporary absence of light? You surely cannot expect to breathe day-air after sunset; your only choice is between the life-giving, health-restoring night-air of the outdoor world and the vitiated, sickening night-air of your sweltering dormitories."

But what the self-torturers are really afraid of is a "draught;" in other words, air in motion. Perceptible currents of air, no matter how pure, no matter how passionately welcomed by the miasma-clogged lungs, they dread as messengers of death. Their fear of night-air is founded chiefly on the circumstance that the cooling of the atmosphere generates air-currents within a few hours after the sunset even of the sultriest day. So they close their bedroom windows or nail them down; they invent double window-sashes and "weather-strips," to exclude the slightest breath of life-air.

And yet the sanitary value of fresh air is generally proportioned to the persistency of its currents. Air in motion removes the impurities of the atmosphere. It renews the supply of oxygen. Its ministrations attend both to the disinfection and the nourishment of the respiratory organs. The sanitary difference between fresh air in motion and stagnant indoor air is that between the pure water of a running fountain and the festering slime of a cesspool.

The comparatively low temperature of night-air only increases its value for expurgative purposes. The appalling, drug-defying mortality of a large city sweltering under the glare of the dog-day sun, is abated by the first spell of cooler weather. The veering of a midsummer breeze from south to northwest reduces the death-rate of infants two-thirds. Canadian trappers who leave their supply-camp with a bad cough, get rid of it on the fifth or sixth day "out." They may get footsore, and if game is scarce, hipped and homesick, but the feeling of haleness about the chest continues. Night-frosts do not affect it. Fatigues rather improve it. They may wake up with a feeling of frost-cramp from their chillblained toes to their shivering knees, but the lungs are at ease; no cough, no asthmatic distress, no stitch-like pains, no night-fever.

An old campaigner would laugh at the idea of "colds" being taken in the open air. He knows that they germinate in close bedrooms and flourish in musty beer-shops, but vanish in the prairie-wind.

Houses cannot be kept too airy, no room or chamber should ever be kept permanently closed for days together. Never mind about the improvement of ventilatory contrivances: patent "ventilators" are mostly calculated to humor the prejudice against perceptible air-currents. They are intended to smuggle in a modicum of fresh air unnoticed, near the edge of the ceiling, in a roundabout way through halls and antechambers. One open window is worth a dozen of such compromise tricks.

Open the dining-room windows in the forenoon; and the kitchen windows in the afternoon; no revolving-fan can compete with the effect of a direct influx of atmospheric air. If you teach a class or work in a warehouse or counting-house, prevail upon the managers to ventilate the place during the dinner-recess; or else try to do your work in the airiest corner, near a window or near the door of an airy hall. In ill-ventilated rooms the azote miasma has its centers of destiny that can be avoided with a little management.

But at all events get rid of the night-air superstition, and enjoy the blessings of an airy bedroom—the luxury, I may add. A natural instinct may be suppressed, but needs but little encouragement to resume its normal functions, like a river returning to its ancient channel. Thus, the fresh-air instinct. In families cursed with the night-air delusion children are often fuddled with miasma till they prefer it to fresh air and dislike to sleep near an open window. But in a single month that aversion can be changed into a decided predilection, till the cool breath of the night- wind becomes a chief condition of a good night's rest, and the closing of the bedroom windows creates a feeling of uneasiness, not unlike the discomfort induced by an attempt to sleep with your head under the blankets. In the sleeping dens of the French village taverns, where after September the window-sashes are actually nailed down, the children of a hygienic home would pine for a draught of oxygen as a sweltering traveler thirsts after fresh water.

Besides open windows, Dio Lewis recommends an open fireplace and a good wood fire all night; but that is a matter of taste; an extra blanket will serve the same purpose, and the danger of damp bed-clothes in mid-winter has been as strangely overrated as the perils of cold drinking-water in midsummer.

In stormy nights a half-closed "rain-shutter" (a window-blind with broad bars) will keep the room perfectly dry without excluding the air. If the mercury sinks below zero, close every window in the house. Intense cold is a disinfectant that purifies even the air of the hide-covered dungeons where the natives of the Polar regions pass the long winter nights.

In the dog-days, on the other hand, do not be satisfied with anything less than a through-draft; open every window in and around the bedroom.

It should also be remembered that the lung-poison of a stifling bed-chamber may undo the sanitary benefit of a long day passed in out-door exercise. European tourists can combine the useful with the agreeable by doing their sightseeing afoot, but should not forget that Alpine morning-breezes may fail to neutralize the bedroom air of a South-German tavern.

Nor can the purest atmosphere of our planet—that of the breezy ocean—be relied upon to counteract the monstrous air-filth of an unventilated cock-pit. Sailors, in spite of an abundance of outdoor exercise, thus often contract lung-disorders, and Captain Cook relates that the natives of the South Sea Islands, after visiting the sailors' cabin of his ship, were seized with strange respiratory afflictions: sneezing-fits, coughs, and pains in the chest, together with a kind of pulmonary fever. Generations of outdoor life had failed to protect these children of Nature against the effects of a brief exposure to a concentrated lung-poison; nay, its effect upon their unprepared organism was more violent than that experienced by persons in whom habit had established a sort of "physiological tolerance"—akin to the strange adaption that enables habitues to swallow enormous doses of arsenic and opium.

For Professor Bates, in his "Naturalist on the River Amazon," states that the natives of Western Brazil have learned by sad experience to avoid a visit to the interior of a white man's dwelling, as travelers in Java would shun the valley of the Upas Tree. Catarrh germs, in their organism, take the form of consumption-microbes, and there appears to be no cure for that disease in the sweltering river swamps of the tropics. The stricken native coughs night and day, and the disease in that virulent modification of its development, terminates life in less than two years. The Quahiba Indians, adds the same traveler, would sooner load the horse of a Caucasian visitor with presents than carry their hospitality to the fatal degree of allowing him to pass a night in their cabins. "Do you bring influenza, Senor?" they ask with a look of alarm, when a stranger approaches their wigwams.

The German, Austrian, and Russian shepherds stay the whole summer with their flocks, but as a class, are nevertheless remarkably subject to pulmonary diseases, and for the following reason: They pass the night in a Schaeferhuette, a sort of ambulance-box, eight feet by four, and six feet high, without windows, but with a tight-fitting sliding door. This door the ill-advised proprietor shuts after dark, and breathes all night the azotized air of his Black Hole of Calcutta on wheels. In the morning he awakens with a hacking cough, superadded to profuse perspiration, and a feeling of nausea. The air of the mountains gradually relieves the other symptoms, but not the cough, which finally becomes chronic. And, with exquisite facilities for the attainment of a patriarchal longevity, the slave of the night-air superstition thus dies in the forenoon of his life.

Cold baths—in air or water—and thorough ventilation become more necessary with every degree further south, and a Spanish army-surgeon of Santiago de Cuba a few years ago surprised the medical faculty with the success of his experiments in the artificial refrigeration of a military hospital. By means of ice-vaults and force-ventilators he cooled some of the wards to a temperature of fifty degrees Fahrenheit below that of the outdoor atmosphere, and cured not only sleeplessness and nervous prostration, but climatic fevers of all sorts, and even cholera. In the treatment of yellow fever his treatment reduced the usual death-rate four-fifths, and that in spite of the fact that his wards were overcrowded and handicapped by the lack of trained nurses.

Practical arguments of that sort will ultimately prevail against prejudice, and it may be safely predicted that hydropathic prescriptions are destined to supersede drug-mongery in the treatment of all germ-diseases, and that before the end of the present century our dwelling-houses will be artificially cooled in summer as successfully as we now warm them in winter.

III - EXERCISE
CHAPTER XI
PHYSIOLOGICAL DATA

The sanitary influence of active exercise is so unmistakable that it has never been altogether disputed, though its importance is still strangely underrated.

Nearly two thousand years ago the medical philosopher Asclepiades substituted gymnastics for drugs, and Dr. Boerhave repeatedly called attention to the remedial effect of outdoor labor in cases where medicine had failed to bring relief. "When I reflect on the pathological immunities of hard-working people," he says, "I cannot help thinking that most of our fashionable diseases might be cured mechanically, instead of chemically, by climbing a bitter-wood tree, or chopping it down, if you like, rather than swallowing a decoction of its disgusting leaves."

The organism of the human body has, indeed, been aptly compared to a vessel moved both by steam and sails, but still more closely resembles the ingenious motor-boat of a Belgian engineer who utilized air-currents to recharge the batteries of an electric propeller. In a calm the ship could for a while continue its course with the assistance of the stored-up power, but under the impulse of a good breeze the engines worked under high pressure, besides being aided by a number of sails. Even thus the activity of the internal organism can for a time dispense with the stimulus of well-directed exercise, but manifests the potency of its assistance with a promptness that precludes all reasonable doubt about the connection of cause and effect. Exposure to a blood-chilling atmosphere makes the generation of animal warmth a question of vital importance, and ten minutes of vigorous exercise will raise that warmth from twenty to thirty degrees. Picket-posts on the Manitoba frontier often keep themselves alive by running, instead of walking, up and clown, for half-hours or longer. Premier Gladstone's prescription of "a cord of beechwood a week, axe and wedges, in six instalments, before breakfast," will stimulate the appetite in a manner which no drugs can begin to approach.

Walking up a hill of two hundred feet suffices to increase the pulse and relieve oppression of the chest and other premonitory symptoms of heart-disease. Sleeplessness can be cured, or rather palliated, by narcotics—for a while. The eventual effect of the drug is to aggravate the evil and induce those fifty-hour vigils that drove De Quincey to the verge of insanity. Outdoor exercise will remedy the trouble, not only more cheaply and reliably, but also without the risk of distressing after-effects.

Skilful sailors can utilize any—not too violent—breeze, to keep their course in the desired direction, and there is hardly a form of active exercise that cannot be modified in a manner to obviate the necessity of the drug-monger's assistance, but, besides, there are movement-cure prescriptions of a more limited, but also more infallible efficacy, that may ultimately supersede the use of medicinal specifics.

CHAPTER XII
OUTDOOR EXERCISE

The principles of regeneration by natural hygiene may be summed up in Dr. Hufeland's advice, to "re-establish, as far as practicable, the conditions to which our organism became adapted during the infinite series of ages preceding the era of indoor-life and made-dishes." The human constitution—physical and moral—was never intended for the sloth of the domestic habits enforced by our sabbatharian civilization. Man's predecessors in the scale of organic evolution were the most restlessly active of all vertebrate animals. Our Darwinian cousins pass their life in the gymnasia of nature—the tree-tops of the tropical virgin-woods; their meals, courtships, and forays alternate with acrobatic exploits; they build no nests; except an occasional rain-shelter, and carry their young in their migrations from forest to forest.

Almost equally active, and even more athletic, man-like creatures inhabited this planet for a period variously estimated from 25,000 to half a million years. Human skeletons have been found among the strata of former geological ages and associated with the bones of such prehistoric animals as mammoths and cave-bears. They were tree-climbers and tree-food eaters, at first, those semi-human progenitors of ours, and in their encounters with the giant-cats of the tropics developed that dread of darkness and night-hags still haunting our mental condition, with all its instinctive love of forest-life. Venturing further and further from their equatorial birthlands, our primitive ancestors became hunters; then nomadic herders, and finally stock-farmers, trying their luck with various methods of agriculture.

During that infinite series of generations the beings that evolved our organism may have strayed into strange forms of idolatry and refuted the belief in the universality of moral institutions; but they certainly did not fail to worship the goddess of health in her own temples. They were runners, swimmers, leapers, hill-climbers, wrestlers, boxers. and spearmen; outdoor exercise yielded them both the means of life and the opportunities for recreation. And it would be a mistake to suppose that the brief era of indoor life had modified our physical constitution in any essential respect. Rivers run most easily in their ancient channels. Remedy-mongers have tried the effect of concentrated food—pure fat, sugar, albumen, and so forth, but it was found that the human stomach preferred more concrete substances. "Whole-wheat bread." with all its innutritive admixtures, is more digestible than pure starch.

Chemically the reason why is not quite clear, but we may suspect that it has a good deal to do with habits formed during the long ages preceding the advent of Liebig's food extracts.

And Nature declines to ratify the contract of kid-gloved brain-workers with the inventors of labor-saving machinery. Intellectual development, to be sure, is the quintescence of all that distinguishes man from his brute fellow- creatures; but beings of our species cannot thrive on metaphysics alone, any more than on Dr. Bernard's Elixir of Life. To avoid dyspepsia, insomnia, hemorrhoids, and sick headaches the Trismegistus of Science has now and then to descend from his study and exercise his motive muscles in the playgrounds of the hirsute anthropoids. Dr. Boerhave's remark that we ought to substitute mechanical for chemical remedies has been paraphrased in the apothegm that "patients might walk away from a good many diseases." Pedestrianism is, indeed, the readiest of all forms of active exercise—doubly effective to burden-carriers, though a health-seeker need not take up his whole bed to walk. A stout overcoat in winter and a market-basket in summer are enough to outweigh the influence of habit which in the course of years might otherwise modify the efficiency of the prescription. An old physician of my acquaintance often repeats his assertion that the best advice a doctor could give to a friend (as distinct from a fee-paying patient) would be to choose his dwelling on some out-of-the-way hill-top, or similar location, at a safe distance from the temptation of the street-car lines, and to readopt the good old democratic habit of doing his own shopping.

"Where street-cars reach," he says, "there will be always a pretext for using them, in spite of solemn pledges to the contrary. It will be storms in winter and heat in summer, or special hurry, where meteorological excuses fail. But in the form of Hobson's choice an excellent movement-cure remedy will get a chance to prove itsefficacy. The walking-habit may ruin a dozen extra pair of shoes per year, and the random shopper is apt to fare worse than the patron of a grocery-wagon; but he is sure to bring home a cargo of health."

A keen appetite for supper, for instance, and a fair chance for a good night's rest. The effect of pedestrianism as a specific for the cure of insomnia can be tested by the simple plan of an occasional intermission. A stay-at-home day being pretty sure to be followed by twice the usual number of sleepless hours.

The organs of the human body are weakened by disuse and invigorated by active service; unexercised muscles become flabby, teeth decay upon a diet of pap; our very hair dies and drops like dead leaves if the constant wearing of hats and night-caps makes it superfluous. And to a quite unsuspected degree the same holds good of our respiratory organs. Exercise that makes the lungs work to the limit of their capacity tends to gradually enlarge that limit. Consumptives not too far advanced toward the stage of total collapse may purchase a new lease of life by exercise stimulating the action of the torpid lungs. A few years ago an emaciated Canadian miner came South for his health and located a small placer claim on the plateau of "Fort Mountain" in Murray County, Georgia. The mountain is a mile high—a cloud-capped outpost of the Southern Alleghanies, and the up-trip, with a few dozen eggs from the next valley farm, obliged the miner to stop every few minutes to keep his chest from bursting; but before the end of the year he was able to make the same trip, without a stop, with a bushel-bag full of cornmeal. The waste from the ravages of the tubercle microbes can perhaps never be repaired but the healthy tissue of the remaining portion of the lung is susceptible both of expansion and invigoration. The lungs expand and contract with the chest.

If three sisters marry on the same day—the first a ferryman, and learns to row a boat; the second a tailor and takes to tight lacing; the third a grocer and tends his shop, an autopsy would show that in twenty years after their separation the ferrywoman's lungs have grown fifty per cent. larger than the shopkeeper's and fully twice as large as the dressmaker's.

"Health is the chief of all earthly blessings," Lord Chesterfield writes to his son;" so much so, indeed, that a healthy beggar is happier than a bedridden king; and the only way in which a rich man can avoid the forfeiture of his birthright to happiness is to live as frugally and laboriously as if he were poor."

Still, strenuous exercise may to a considerable degree atone for dietetic indulgences, and few observers of men and habits can fail to have noticed Epicureans whom a sort of instinct prompts to give themselves the benefit of a movement-cure—stout, florid gormands who decline to become torpid, and walk habitually at a double-quick or go out of their w\ay to join in athletic sports. The net result in happiness may not get them above the average by that method; but they keep disease at bay:

"Lass nach Riesen-Kraft ihn streben, Wer im Uebermass geniesst; Dem Athleten wird vergeben, Was der Schwachling treuer busst." "He would enjoy himself to an excessive degree should likewise try to exceed in vigor; an athlete may take risks that might prove fatal to a weakling."

A considerable help to such endeavors in muscular Christianity is the possession of a little real estate, an orchard or patch of truck-farm, that can be worked for a practical purpose and with visible results. Uncle Toby, in digging up his brother's kitchen-garden to illustrate the Vauban system of ramparts, incidentally also erected fortifications against the inroads of decrepitude, and it has been repeatedly observed that individuals who attained to an extreme old age were generally (like Jenkins, Darapsky, and Thomas Parr) poor rustics whose avocations required daily labor in the fields and woods. The German foresters, or wardens of government woodlands, are likewise longlived, with the noteworthy exception of aristocrats who enter a Forst-schule (College of Forestry) in reliance on family influence and rapid promotion, and really most of them contrive to get hold of a sinecure, enabling them to earn a high salary by a few hours of office-work, or retire on a liberal pension. But their lease of life is equally limited, while the poor Revier Foerster who has to plant some threescore saplings every week-day, has a first-class chance to continue his ministrations for as many years.

For the same reason school-trustees should strain the limits of their tolerance, rather than discourage the passion for out-door sports that distinguishes the youngsters of the progressive nations from the whelps of decadence. Football, baseball, aquatic sports, and the "Hare and Hound "races of the British colleges, serve a purpose of moral as well as physical sanitation, for some of the besetting vices of youth are symptoms of abnormal physical inactivity—effects, in fact, as often as causes of disease.

No clamor for outing-sports interfere with the curriculum of South-European colleges, and that fact is far more ominous than the alleged tendency to rowdyism that alarms old women of both sexes in our Northern university towns. The civilization of Greece and Moorish Spain sprang from barbarism like water from the rock in the desert of Sinai, while physical indolence is the torpor that precedes the collapse of moribund nations, and heralds a moral night that knows no morning.

CHAPTER XIII
INDOOR EXERCISE

In latitudes of an inhospitable climate an opportunity for indoor exercise has indisputable advantages, but involves the risk of defective ventilation, and the ideal of a rainday refuge for votaries of the movement-cure is the drill-shed of an Austrian household regiment: A structure 300 feet long by 60 broad, and about 25 feet between the floor and the ceiling of the main hall, yet equipped with hot-air pipes sufficient to counteract the frosts of the coldest winter day.

A time may come when every country town of the civilized North-lands will have a public gymnasium of that sort, and in the meanwhile in door-workers must contrive to defy the main obstacle to effective ventilation, viz., the superstitious dread of cold draughts.

The supposed connection of catarrhs ("colds") with currents of cold air is strikingly refuted by the practical argument of an open smithy. Blacksmith—as well as the operatives of Northern rolling-mills—often work all day long in close proximity to a blazing fire, while a wide-open door admits the blizzards of the midwinter season; yes their health and longevity is far above the average and might rank with that of gardeners, if they were not obliged to inhale coal-fumes, as well as ice-winds. Their special work, it is true, tends to counteract the effects of the onesided system of exercise that explains the shortcomings of nine out of ten health-seekers. "Our patients get an immense deal of encouragement to develop the muscles of their motive organs," \\ritcs the visitor of a climatic sanitarium;" there are mountain-excursions and forest-excursions, five times a week, and every evening troops of volunteers clamber up a prospect rock to see the sunset and get an appetite for supper. Besides, there is a Kneipp-cure department, and the trots through the wet meadow often take the form of a footrace. But what are our arms doing all that while? Lifting a half-ounce spoon from plate to mouth or reaching up to take a hat from the rack."

It would be no exaggeration to say that the legs of the average city dweller get a thousand times as much exercise as his arms.

Amateur-blacksmithing, on the Elihu Burritt plan, remedies that disproportion, and the "Learned Blacksmith" went so far as to recommend it as a mental and moral remedy. He learned to speak four different languages and had a book acquaintance with half a dozen more, including Hebrew and Greek. Memorizing a hundred words an hour was about the average of his linguistic tasks, up to his fiftieth year, and he was firmly persuaded that sledgehammer matinee helped to counterbalance the deadweight of such burdens. And, moreover, he considered a visit to his smithy a ready expedient in ethical emergencies. If anything happened to rouse his indignation he would skip downstair and hammer away like Thor and Vulcan for a minute or two, then draw a deep breath and feel that the rising choler had been successfully "worked off." "What else would you propose?" he inquires; "sit still and swallow your wrath, to imitate the saints? Well, try it, and see if the suppressed gall doesn't surge back a dozen times before night, making you as cross as an old spinster with no moral outlet but her scandalous tongue."

Sledge-hammering also helps to invigorate the lungs and shake the diaphragm in a manner pretty sure to dislodge the lurking imps of dyspepsia. Violent movement-cures may not be advisable in the far-gone stages of debilitating disorders, but, on the whole, will do for a crapulent organism what a brisk gale does for the forests of a tropical coast-swamp that may vegetate in a calm, but cannot get rid of their dead leaves and mouldering branches. Microbes have a predilection for a quiet boarding-house and do not often frequent a blacksmith's body.

Woodchopping answers the same purpose, and in a climate like that of our lake-shore States it would be worth while to weather-tighten and warm a shed, in order to try Mr. Gladstone's favorite prescription without the risk of frozen toes. The "Sage of Hawarclen" worked in the open air, but the winter-climate of Southern Britain, under the parallel of Montreal, is in reality milder than that of Maryland. Wood-choppers indulging the luxury of a weatherproof building— heated, perhaps, with a chip-fire flickering in an open fireplace, can now and then give their lungs the benefit of a draught of purer oxygen by stepping out in the storm and fetching additional logs from the woodpile.

Asthma-patients, with a little experience in the caprices of their mysterious disorder, will not be apt to protract that special test of strength beyond the first premonitions of fatigue. Burden-carrying is always liable to bring on a spasmodic fit of an affection that cannot be provoked by other forms of exercise, even in preposterous overdoses. A bicyclist may work his pedals till his spine is twisted by cramps and his fingers threaten to relax their grip; his lungs may heave and gasp without betraying any other symptoms of distress, a pedestrian may trudge along till his knee-joints stagger and sleep tries to enforce its rights in the middle of the track, but no trace of asthma, while a shouldered weight of perhaps less than a hundred pounds suddenly "cuts the breath," as if the valves of the respira-tory apparatus had closed with a snap. "Dyspnoea," or air-famine, pathologists call a paroxysm of that sort, and the difficulty in drawing a full breath may yield to a cold sponge-bath or defy all remedies and keep the patient in misery for weeks together.

Light indoor work: amateur carpentering, house-cleaning, adjusting stove-pipes or library shelves, is, on the other hand, the most efficient of all asthma-cures, and far more permanent in its effects than the chemical specifics (stramonium smoke, etc.) that relieve the spasm for a few minutes without preventing the risk of a speedy relapse. And it is a curious and almost unaccountable fact that smoke, dust, and other impurities of the indoor atmosphere, rather enhance the effectiveness of the prescription for that special purpose. The most plausible guess at the rationale of that experience is the conjecture that the aforesaid admixtures of the indoor air oblige the lungs to effect the \\ork of expulsion by opening some gate which incidentally relieves the spasm of the asthma-fit. Always provided that the remedy is applied only at long intervals and in moderate doses. An excess of dust, breathed day after day, clogs the tissue of the lungs to an irremediable degree, and millers are notoriously subject to chronic asthma in its most incurable. if not most distressing, forms.

The poet-philosopher Goethe remarks that every brain-worker should consult his sanitary interests by following some mechanical trade as a by-occupation, and the successor of Frederic the Great made that advice a pretext for establishing the rule that every prince of the House of Prussia must serve an apprenticeship at some handicraft. Some of the uniformed youngsters accordingly learn printing, others bookbinding, but about four out of five prefer a curriculum in a carpenter's shop. A hundred years ago the Berlin wits used to hint that the by-law in question might prove useful under circumstances that obliged a good many refugees from neighboring France to try their hands at the unaccustomed occupation of useful work, but the rule is still in force, and none of the royal blue-coats have been the worse for the investiture of a carpenter's apron. Joiner's work: sawing, jack-planing, and hammering exercises nearly every muscle of the human body, and has the incidental advantage of a pastime that grows on the habit and can become a passion, like gardening and watchmaking.

And not all "exercise with a useful by-purpose" can be recommended from that point of view. There are some extremely utilitarian occupations that lack the spice of variety and a personal interest. In some cities of British India, where labor is cheap and coal very dear, hundreds of vagabonds are often roped in to operate the machinery of a large workshop on the treadmill plan; but in spite of sanitary precautions a wheel-treader every now and then steps down and out with the unfeigned symptoms of complete exhaustion. "I tried it, for the fun of it," says Sir Samuel Baker, "but was unable to persist for more than ten minutes, though I am pretty sure that in my Ceylonese mountain camp the excitement of a boar-chase often enabled me to exert the tenfold amount of muscular effort without any conscious trace of fatigue."

Every well-arranged household, in fact, should have an indoor sanitarium in the form of a general repair-shop, or Jack-of-all-trades resort. From an artistic point of view the products of the establishment may prove shameful failures, but they will save doctor's bills and perhaps police-court fines.

" In freeing themselves from the bonds of an unworthy attachment," says Madame de Sevigne, "men have one great advantage: they can plunge into business, and forget;"—and a rush into a convenient workshop will often solve the problem of fighting clown minor temptations that cannot be exorcised by study.

Combined with wholesome food and steady habits, indoor work has more than once enabled city-dwellers to emulate the physical prowess of rustics. Frederic Barbarossa's armies had been recruited among the bare-fisted peasantry of the South-German highlands but on the battlefield of Legano were crushingly defeated by the trainbands of some fourteen Italian cities. Roman legionaries held their own against the giants of the Teutonic forests, and the levies of the Hanseatic League prevailed against the federation of the iron-clad cavaliers that had for centuries treated them as an inferior species of bipeds. Lionheart Richard came to grief in a siege, and his German peer, Eberhart Longbeard of Wirtemberg was terribly beaten by the home-guards of a little manufacturing town.

"Wie haben da die Gerber so meisterlich gegerbt;

Wie haben da die Farber so blutig roth gefarbt"— "How the tanners plied their trade, How the dyers dyed so red!"

—and all that in spite of the fact that the artisans of the Middle Ages were physically handicapped by the unsanitary condition of their streets and dwellings.

CHAPTER XIV

GYMNASTICS

Primitive nations can dispense with physical training-schools as the creatures of the wilderness dispense with houses and clothes, but city-dwellers need a substitute for the lost opportunities of outdoor exercise. Mental culture and gymnastics should be as inseparable as body and soul. "It is impossible to repress luxury by legislation," says Solon in Lucian's "Dialogues of Anacharsis," but its influence may be counteracted by athletic games, which invigorate the body and give a martial character to the amusements of our young men."

And that remedial use of gymnastics requires the supervision of an expert teacher. It is not enough to provide an assortment of training-school apparatus and trust visitors to use it to good advantage. We might as well establish a free public drug-store and invite patients to come in and help themselves. I have seen athletics on the Let-Alone plan tried in a city park, and remember the results in the case of novices who got discouraged the first day by disfiguring accidents, and of others who contracted dyspepsia by exercising directly after dinner.

A well-developed system of physical culture offers remedies for almost even disorder of the human organism, and for all but the most hopeless malformations.

As a preliminary, gymnasium pupils should be advised to postpone the principal meal of the day (call it supper or dinner) to the late afternoon, and at least half an hour after the conclusion of their exercises. Violent muscular efforts can exhaust the vital vigor of the organism to a degree which—for a short time—may take away the appetite, and make it advisable to defer repletion for a little while; but even a direct rush from the gymnasium to the dining- room would be hygienically preferable to the opposite mistake.

After-dinner rest is recommended by the plainest monitions of instinct, by drowsiness, apathy, and aversion to strenuous efforts of any kind. After being nursed, a fretful child will fall asleep; gorged animals become torpid and retire to a resting-place—some of them for days and weeks. The physiological reason can be found in the fact that exercise interferes with digestion, and obliges the stomach to retain an accumulation of ingesta till there is a risk of their undergoing a process of fermentation and becoming a positive danger to the system they were intended to nourish.

Beginners should also be warned against the mistake of continuing any special exercise to the length of excessive fatigue, and to avoid debilitating perspiration by choosing the lightest dress compatible with decency and comfort. "Gym-nos," in the language of the ancient champion gymnasts, meant "naked." A hampering load of drygoods is, indeed, often the first impediment to the free use of our motive organs, and the professional English trainer Stephens, of sprinting fame, recorded his experience that barefoot boys were his most promising pupils, because perfectly straight toes are of primary importance as qualifications for a victory on the footrace course.

The kittels of South-German schoolboys—jackets with sleeves terminating at the elbow—are hard to beat for gymnastic purposes; and on general sanitary principles a course of physical culture should begin with arm- exercises. Dr. Schrodt called attention to the fact that in newborn children the lower extremities are only slightly larger than the arms, and that in our nearest zoological relatives the difference is next to nothing. But from the first to the end of the fourteenth year, when a boy may chance to be apprenticed to a handicraft, his legs get about ten times as many opportunities for development. At every step the muscles of the lower motive organs have to lift and move the weight of the body, while his hands are pocketed for future reference or swing idly to and fro. The result is a partial and unsymmetric tendency of growth. The stout pedestals of the organism support a rickety superstructure.

It should be the first object of gymnastics to counteract the consequences of that mistake, and a disposition to pulmonary disorders can thus often be nipped in the germ. Microbes are especially apt to fasten upon torpid and neglected parts of the organism. Like caterpillars scattered by a gale, they can be dislodged by a movement-cure, and, besides, arm-gymnastics help to correct the most frequent of all malformations: vis., a narrow chest.

Weak lungs must have been a rarely-heard-of complaint at a time when the rising generation of a whole continent was trained in spear-throwing. Consumption microbes had no chance to effect a lodging in a body getting the benefit of that exercise. And as a prescription for the lung-suffering results of indoor life no remedy of the drugstore can compete with a course of Gerwerfen, as the German turners call their attempt to revise that form of athletics, which a modern educator describes as follows:

"The missile is a lance of some tough wood (ash and hickory preferred) about ten feet long and one and a half inches in diameter, terminating in a blunt iron knob to steady the throw and keep the wood from splintering. A heavy post with a movable top-piece (the Ger-block) forms the target, the head-shaped top being secured by means of a stout cramp-hinge that permits it to turn over, but not to fall down. Distance all the way from ten to forty paces Grasp the spear near the middle, raise it to the height of your ear, plant the left foot firmly on the ground, the right knee slightly bent, fix your eye on the target, lean back and let drive. If you hit the log squarely in the center, or a trifle higher up, it will topple over, but, still hanging by the clasp-hinge, can be quickly adjusted for the next thrower. A feeble hit will not stir the ponderous Ger-block; the spear has to impinge with the force of a sixty- pound blow, so that a successful throw is also an athletic triumph. The German spear throwers are generally lads after the heart of Charles Reade—ambidextrous boys, whose either handed strength and skill illustrates the fact that the antiquity of a prejudice proves nothing in its favor." For indoor exercise an equivalent can be constructed with a stout rope and a couple of leather-covered iron rings—say, six inches in diameter. Dangling from a high ceiling or the beam of a barn, a grapple-swing can be used for a great variety of acrobatic evolutions: Dangling, swinging to and fro, slowly at first, then faster and faster (with the aid of the plunging feet); "turning over," and whirling heels over head, till the protest of the wrist-joints enforces a pause.

Breathing-pauses will be often needed the first week, but afterwards at even longer intervals—indicating the lung-strengthening effects of the exercise.

Lifting weights and holding them out at arm's length is a favorite amusement of the Tyrolese peasants, whose knee-joints mountain climbing has made almost fatigue-proof, and who intuitively seem to recognize the expedience of giving their arms the benefit of a movement cure. A by-purpose of theirs is the wish to strengthen their wrists for the ordeal of a wrestling match, and wrestlers with the incubus of a hereditary disorder would often do well to imitate their example.

Weight lifting in that manner is the germ of the dumb-bell cure and in more than one sense the hardiest of all health exercises. A homemade sandbag or a pail full of water will do for a beginning. In rain-weather, when the programme for pedestrian exercise has to be cancelled, dumb-bells or their substitutes are still available, even in a tenement attic, and their persistent use can be guaranteed to redeem the victims of general debility.

The beneficial effects of the exercise are indeed almost sure to manifest themselves in time to obviate the most of all pathological risks: The moral collapse of a patient who resigns himself to his fate and plunges into dissipations to "make an end of it" and harden the consummation of what he has come to consider an inevitable doom. A Texas cotton planter of my acquaintance worked like a beaver to save his crop from a protracted drought, but after watching the signs of the sky day after day for two months and seeing no indication of a change, all of a sudden became reckless, sold his horses, harness and farming tools at throw-away prices, got drunk, and wound up with an escapade that obliged him to enlist in the army to have a tent, if not a roof, over his head. A week after that cataclysm of his hopes the long-prayed for rain-clouds did rise from the gulf, and a series of abundant showers enabled the purchaser of his farm to double his stake the first year.

"Blast such a climate," growled his predecessor in self-defence, "if there had been the least sign of a change a little sooner, I might have pulled through."

And in that respect remedial gymnastics offer an inestimable advantage, both over drug-mongery and all sorts of faith-cures.

There are ebbs and tides in the vicissitudes of vital vigor, and the self-regulating faculties of the organism may rally in a manner to overcome both the disease and the drug; abiding faith may at last reward the patron of a prayer agent. But in either case the hoped-for symptoms of recovery are sadly apt to reveal themselves too late—the normal tendency of the experiment being, indeed, a change from bad to worse, for the sweat-box misery of a prayer conclave may prove as baneful as a course of blue-pills. Peering desperately for a sign of dawn, the patient at last becomes impatient, and procures an anodyne, or takes other measures to travel the dark road as swiftly as possible.

Movement-cures, on the other hand, reveal their benefit after the end of a week or so—at first by improvements in the facility of the exercise itself, but soon also by indisputable physiological changes for the better. The appetite revives, sleep becomes quieter and more protracted, till the depressing feeling of helplessness gives way to the buoyancy of self-confidence.

In that way Dr. Winship of Boston recovered his lost self-respect. The "crime of weakness" had obliged him to submit to the insults of a bully, and he resolved to become a man in the ancient heroic sense of the word or renounce an existence whose blessings had ceased to outweigh its evils. Lifting weights and swinging a pair of ring- weighted Indian clubs soon began to improve his appearance and inspire him with hopes he would not have bartered the wealth of a sick boodle magnate, but he continued his exercises, adding heavier and heavier rings, he continued to throw weights and lift weights till he became the physical superior of his insulter and at last a modern Samson, able to handle burdens in a way that transcends belief—and incidentally equally expert in the task of grappling with the burdens of existence. Bag-punching may be made a diverting intermezzo of more strenuous exercises, and it is altogether a good plan to vary the programme of gymnastic prescriptions, now and then. There, as elsewhere, a change of employment will make frequent fast days less necessary. Canadian lumbermen, in the blest absence of Blue-law spies, often devote their Sundays to hunting trips and scramble up and down deep mountain ridges, with all the energy of sportsmen who have passed the week in a city office and need their holidays for outdoor exercise. Those anti-Sabbatharian woodcutters may actually get a double dose of hard work on their leisure day, but cheerfully go to chopping again on Monday morning, while a month of uniform drudgery would probably put half of them on the sick-list. That there are true specifics on the remedy-list of the gymnasium, as well as of the drug store, is proved by the efficacy of the movement-cure for asthma. A straight stick, about five feet long, is marked from end to end with deep notches—some twenty of them altogether. A ten-pound weight with a hook complete the inexpensive apparatus. The exercise consists in grasping the stick at the thicker end, raising it to the level of the chin and thrusting it out like a fencing-foil, draw it back slowly and push it out again, keeping it as nearly as possible horizontal. Then hook the weight to one of the near-by notches and try to repeat the home- thrust manoeuvre. Every notch further out will increase the weight and the strain on the arm muscles, till at last a slip from the level indicates the limit of the experiment. With the weight on the farthest practicable notch even an athlete will notice that the exercise reacts on the mechanism of the lungs. The breath comes and goes in gasps,— involving coughs, perhaps, if the bronchial tubes are clogged with phlegm, but at the same time the feeling of pulmonary impediments is gradually relieved. The experimenter finds that he can breathe freer and deeper than before. That improvement may not be a permanent one, but the beneficial after-effects of the exercise just suffice to break the spell of an asthma fit. A daily repetition of the cure at last obviates the risk of a relapse for weeks to come; the patient can relax the strictness of his dietetic precaution and venture to leave his sleeping chair for a horizontal couch without the dread of being waked by a suffocation fit.

And it is a significant fact that not every kind of arm-exercise will serve the purpose of an asthma cure. Wood-cutting, for instance, is very apt to exert an opposite effect; the shock seems to aggravate the distress of the lungs and tighten the grip of the dyspnoea or chronic disability to get a full breath of life-air. Nor is that experience limited to weaklings. I remember an interview with a broad-shouldered, but financially rather straightened, Tennessee mountain carpenter, who confessed with a sigh that he was obliged to do nearly all his axe work by proxy. "I used to try it, anyhow," said he, "but it 'cut my wind' so often that I'm not going to put my foot in that trap again. It's better to be poor than going through such misery"—stating several cases to illustrate a theory to the effect that fate had reduced him to the alternative of getting short of cash or of air. Weight-carrying in warm weather, by the way, is likewise so unmistakably detrimental to the comfort of weak lungs, that asthma patients instinctively avoid farm work, though they may be fond of country life and outdoor exercise.

About twenty years ago a North Yankee invented a "rowing machine," which he intended to facilitate the preparatory exercises of oarsmen,—without perhaps suspecting that he had provided an almost infallible mechanical constipation cure. The apparatus can be worked indoors, and adapted to various degrees of strength, and the exercise (a close imitation of the movements incident to the task of rowing a cockle-boat against the stream) reacts on the functions of the digestive organs in a manner that must be experienced to be credited. Close tools that have resisted other sanitary prescriptions and yielded only temporarily to drastic drugs, are relieved permanently before the end of half a week. An hour of work in the morning and about half an hour in the evening (before supper) is enough to insure that result, and in combination with cold sponge-baths will make drug-medication wholly superfluous in all but the most inveterate cases of dyspepsia. Far-gone dyspeptics have to invoke the third remedy of nature: A fasting-cure. In cool weather the triple prescription will do its work in a couple of weeks and so effectively that subsequent relapses can be avoided by the most ordinary dietetic precautions.

In a former chapter I have mentioned a movement-cure specific for diarrhoea, viz., pedestrian exercise, especially in warm weather. On stormy winter days carrying weights (say, buckets full of coal) upstairs, for an hour or two, will prove a remedial equivalent. With the co-operation of a spare diet its efficacy will manifest itself before the end of the second day, unless the digestive organs should have been outrageously deranged by the abuse of virulent drugs.

Sleeplessness will eventually yield to almost any kind of physical exercise (quicker than to brain work), but among its mechanical specifics a German physician mentions mountain climbing. In explanation of his personal experience he has a theory that vertigo (dizziness) and the excitement of a perilous path at the brink of steep cliffs affect the brain in a manner that craves the relief of sleep. He also recommends several gymnastic substitutes (Ersatz Mittel), e. g., ladder climbing on the hand-over-hand plan. Place a long stout ladder against a wall at an angle of 45 degrees, and attend to the precautions against the risk of slipping. Then step underneath, grasp the highest round you can reach with outstretched arms, draw yourself up to the next higher one—feet now dangling clear off the ground; up to the next, higher again, and so on, till dizziness or exhaustion suggest the descent of man. Rest for a few minutes, or engage in lighter exercise, then at it again, and after half an hour of ups and downs conclude the soiree, and watch its effects on the chance for a good night's rest. It is a common experience of mountain tourists that, upon retiring for the night, they are for a while haunted by visions of yawning chasms, till yawns of a different sort offer a change of programme, and the Brocken-spectre ridden brain seeks refuge in slumber. The blest contrast of the horizontal couch may help to enhance the attractiveness of that change, and sleep supervenes without the aid of opiates.

The excitement of competitive gymnastics is equally effective in relieving the torpor of the reaction following the abuse of strong liquors. With all the firm resolves inspired by the appeals of a temperance orator, the new convert cannot help feeling a more and more urgent craving for a stimulant of some sort or other, and by a sort of instinct, welcomes an opportunity for soul-stirring pastimes. Miners at work in a bonanza pit would scorn the offer of a dram-bottle—they have found a more pleasant intoxicant. Gamblers, too, become abstemious under the influence of an exciting game, especially as long as the dice fall in their favor; and mountain peak climbers of the Tyndall school ask no better tonic.

CHAPTER XV
FREE MOVEMENT CURES OR SANITARIUM EXERCISES

There are health seekers so exhausted by wasting diseases or the abuse of drugs that they are unable to participate in the exercises of a public gymnasium. Old school physicians would have consigned them to the inactivity of a sweltering sick-room. Faith curists, with their antics, would to some degree mitigate the tedium of that ordeal; but the patient would still be doomed to that most grievous trial of patience: the necessity to suffer without a chance to promote the progress of improvement by individual efforts.

The movement cure plan offers that chance even to the most far-gone victims of debilitating disorders. As long as the apathy of exhaustion has not yet merged in the trance of the endless night, the possibility of exercise always implies the possibility of recovery.

The manager of a "Life-under-glass" hospital invited patronage by an artistic signboard, informing the public that "Warmth is Life, Cold is Death." Yes, death to microbes, at all events, commented an apostle of the refrigeration cure, after mentioning a variety of cases where disease germs could be dislodged or killed by a degree of cold which their living boarding house could survive without difficulty and even without discomfort.

"Motion is life, apathy is death," would be a less misleading motto.

Bedridden patients should not be urged to keep quiet when they begin to fret for a chance to exercise their motive organs in some way or other. Faute de mieux, they may be encouraged to sit up in bed, and recline, by turns, or roll from side to side. It will help to keep the blood in circulation and prevent bed-sores and hyponchondria. Any modification of physical exercise, in fact, will extend its beneficial influence to the mind of the patient, and the protracted slumber following fatigue will assist the remedial efforts of nature, and mitigate distress by the balm of oblivion.

The exercises which follow, illustrated by a number of excellent photographs, can be adapted to every degree of convalescence.

Those movements illustrated with dumb-bells can be taken with free hand or with anything that can be grasped conveniently in the hands. There should not be a weight of over two or three pounds in each hand unless inclined to be strong.

Be very careful not to overdo the exercises the first few attempts.

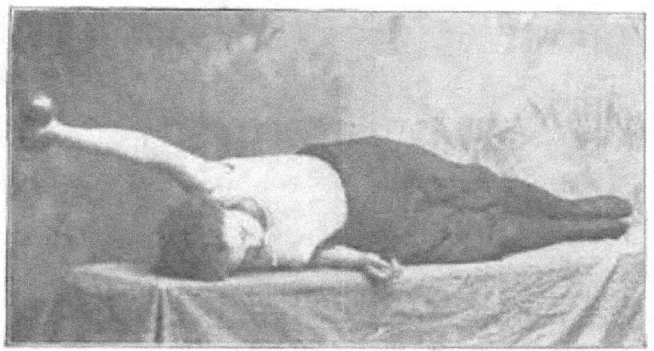

Exercise No. 1 Reclining on right side and raising left arm, with dumb-bell in hand and elbow rigid, from hips to high over head. Same exercise with right arm while reclining on left side. Inhale deep breath as arm goes back.

Exercise No. 1 will relieve the respiratory torpor of debilitating disorders and the aftereffects of pneumonia. Of benefit also in several phases of heart disease.

Exercise No. 2 will aid the functions of the digestive organs and act as a specific in promoting recovery from accidents involving injuries to the spine. Prevented paralysis and greatly relieved the mental distress of the patient in the case

115

of a carpenter who had fallen from a high scaffold and was brought in, pale with terror, and as he supposed permanently crippled in his lower extremities. He had lost the use of his voluntary muscles from the hips down, and felt "numb;" experienced but little benefit from several applications of electricity, but on the fifth day noticed that he could slightly raise one of his feet. Steadily exercising the sinews of that foot, he contrived the next day to raise it about half a yard above the mattress of his bed, and his recovery from that time was continuous and rapid, aided, as it was, by the influence of hope.

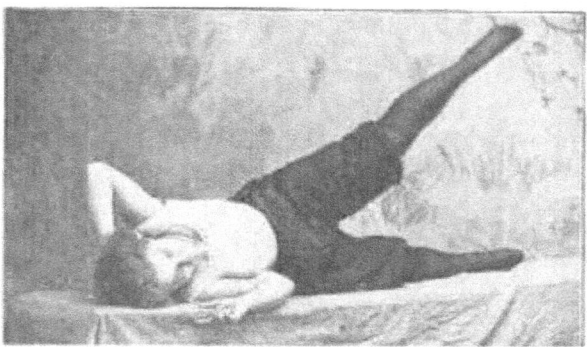

Exercise No 2. Reclining on right side and raising left leg as high as possible and the same exercise taken with right leg while reclining on left side

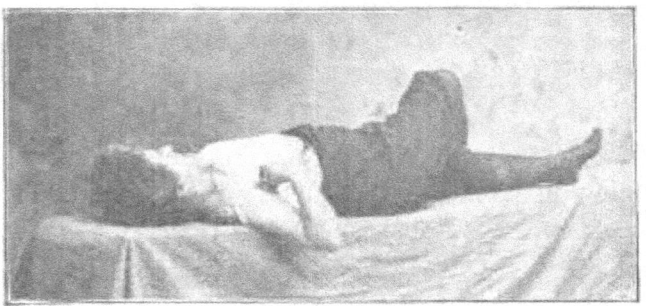

Exercise No. 3. Reclining on back and crossing right leg over left, as far as possible, and vice versa

116

Exercise No. 4 will benefit sufferers from kidney complaints and digestive obstructions. Also an effective remedy for obstructions of the respiratory organs. Its incidental tendency to strengthen the spine should recommend its addition to the list of callisthenics and health movements to be repeated before breakfast every morning in the year.

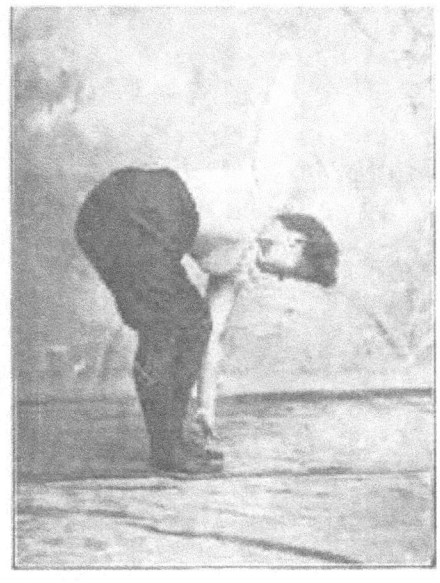

Exercise No. 4. Standing erect, reach and touch the floor, near toe, with left hand, while the right is lifted high over head. Same exercise with position of hands reversed.

Exercise No. 5 is a constipation cure, more permanently effective than any drug, and not followed by troublesome reactions. Combined with cold sponge-baths it will relieve the torpor of the bowels before the evening of the second day. Continue for a quarter of an hour, the first and second morning; for about five minutes every following day. Lengthen or shorten that time according to the varying evidences of efficacy.

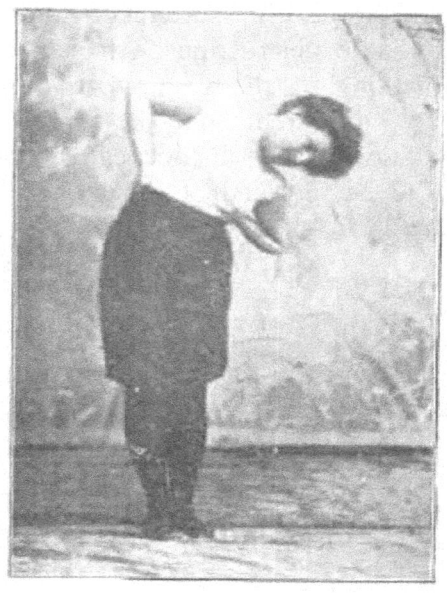

Exercise No. 5, Standing, with hands on hips and knees straight, bending far to the left and right alternately.

Exercise No. 6 is a cure (as well as preventive) for disorders of the kidneys.

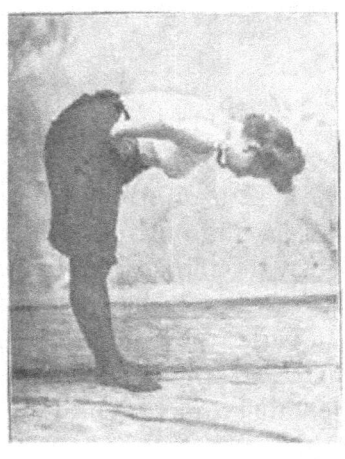

Exercise No. 6, Same position as foregoing, and bending far backward and forward, alternately.

Exercise No. 7 is of advantage in stimulating the actions of the lungs in cases where" patients are unable to leave their bed.

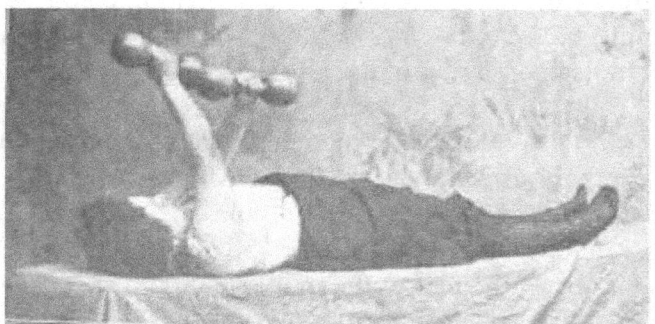

Exercise No. 7. Reclining on back, with dumb-bells in hands at side, raising same with elbows rigid, and crossing arms over chest.

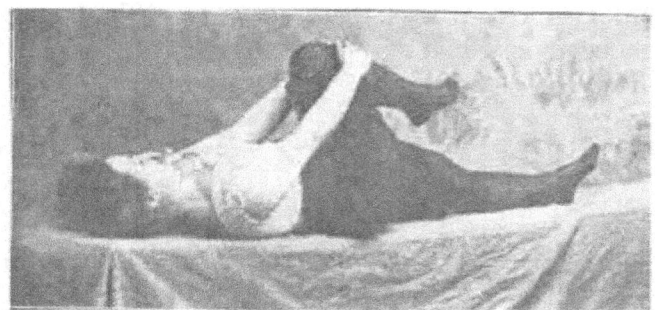

Exercise No. 8. Reclining, bring right leg up, clasping hands over knee and pulling leg up as far as possible.

Exercise No. 8 is a constipation cure for invalids, as well as those desiring to counteract the effects of sedentary occupations. Its adoption in hospitals and sanitariums would obviate the necessity of a resort to laxative drugs.

Exercise No. 9 is an asthma specific. Continued for thirty minutes every evening it will save the patient hours of struggles with agony of suffocation. Like the balance, stick exercise described in the proceeding chapter, it tends to break the spell of the pulmonary spasm, and the danger of a relapse (though extant, as in all phases of the most incalculable of all organic disorders) is not half as

119

imminent as in cases where relief has been obtained by the use of palliating drugs. The fumes of stramonia (Jimson weed, or thorn apple) induce a deadly nausea which, as it were, by the menace of a more serious peril, overcomes the air-famine and sets the lungs a gasping, while the sufferer's face is moistened by a cold perspiration. Inhaling charcoal fumes would provoke similar symptoms. The grip of the choking fit does relax while the nausea lasts, but as soon as the sickening effects of the poison-fumes subside the patient feels the premonitions of pulmonary trouble and hardly ventures to stir for fear of provoking another strangling fit. The effect of the movement cure specific is a relief of a very different kind. The sense of a slight insufficiency in the allowance of life-air still remains, but the lungs move at ease, the obstructive difficulty appears to have been remedied by a direct removal of the cause.

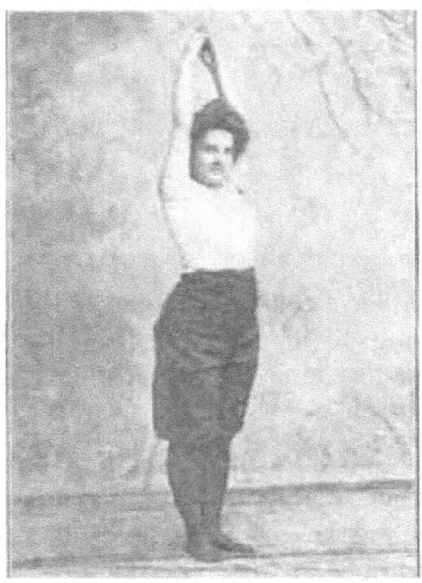

Exercise No. 9. Bringing arms upward and outward from side to position illustrated, and inhaling deep breath and retaining some during the movements.

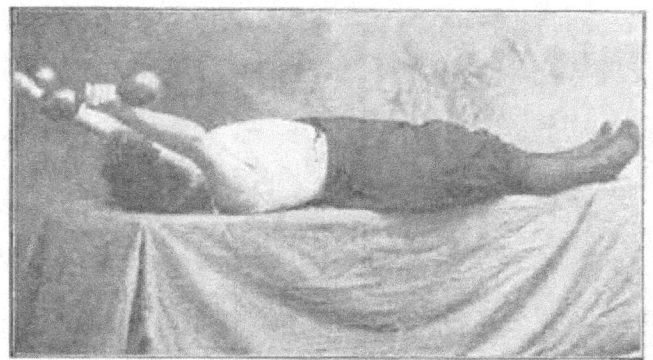

Exercise No. 10. Reclining and bringing arms from far back straight upward with elbows rigid, to straight over chest, drawing deep breath and retaining same during the movement.

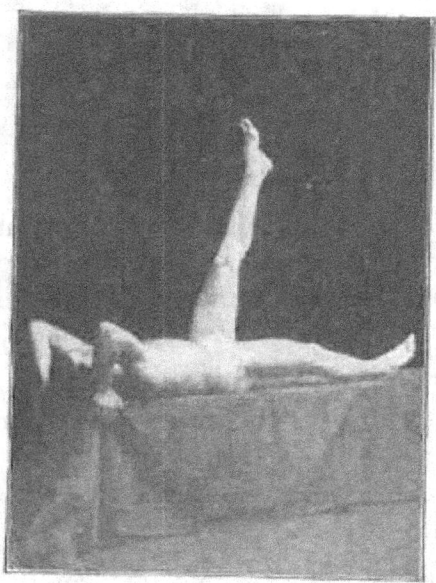

Exercise No. 11. Reclining and raising left leg as high as possible, with knee straight, and repeat same with right leg.

121

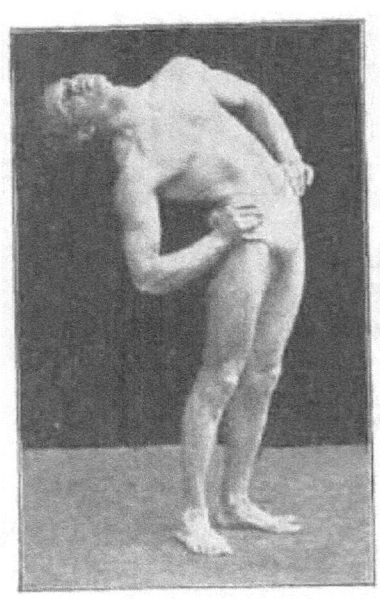

Exercise No. 12. Standing, hands on hips, circulatory body exercise, swinging body in circular manner right, left, back and forward.

Exercise No. 13 is a severe test of the abdominal muscles, but of great benefit to invalids who are temporarily incapacitated from pedestrian exercise, as by injuries to the foot or flexor sinews. May be continued, with long pauses, for a quarter of an hour at a time, twice or three times a day.

Exercise No. 14 is about the best movement to bring relief from the vigor of sinews strained by weight-lifting, or stiffened by long-continued inactivity, as in the case of bedridden invalids.

Exercise No. 15 will strengthen the muscles of the neck and shoulder and might often exceed the efficacy of local application in breaking the spell of tetanus, or "lockjaw." The premonitory symptoms of that mysterious disorder are frequently attended with a feeling of soreness about the very muscles which this form of dumbbell exercise tends to invigorate. "Keep moving your arms, keep moving your arms," was Dr. Benjamin Rush's constant advice to sufferers from injuries that began to threaten tetanic complications.

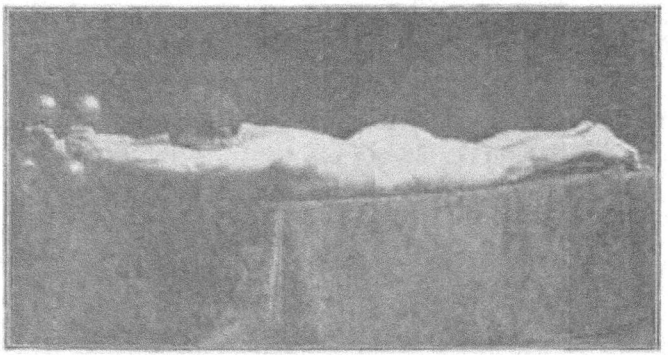

Exercise No 15. Reclining on stomach, grasping dumb bells in hand, raising arms from hanging position to position illustrated

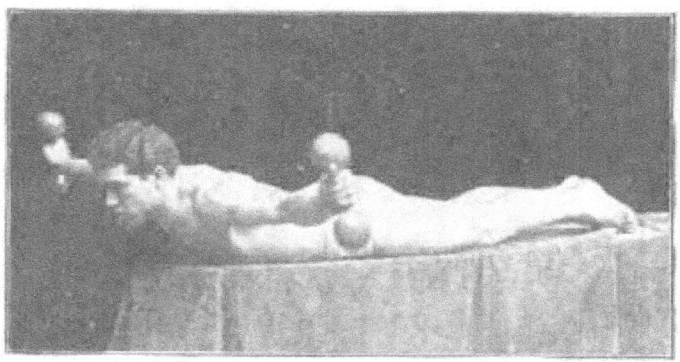

Exercise Nos. 16 and 17. Reclining, arms hanging, raising bells upward and outward from the body, level with shoulders. Reversing that motion by bringing bells from position illustrated as No 15 to position on level

Exercises Nos. 16 and 17 are modifications of the foregoing, and the best "vivacious exercise" for invalids temporarily deprived of the use of their lower extremities. Soldiers with their shoulder-joints cramped by the straps of a heavy knapsack and with their arms hanging idle, can be kept in a fair state of health by pedestrian exercise alone, and, vice versa, the total inactivity of the lower motive organs may be compensated by a persistent use of dumb-bells in the manner described in the two last paragraphs.

Exercise No. 18 is a movement cure for invalids, but also a first-class aid to digestion under circumstances making other forms of exercise unavailable. It is a last resort kind of motion cure and affords a fair chance to test the difference between the simplest sort of exercise and no exercise at all.

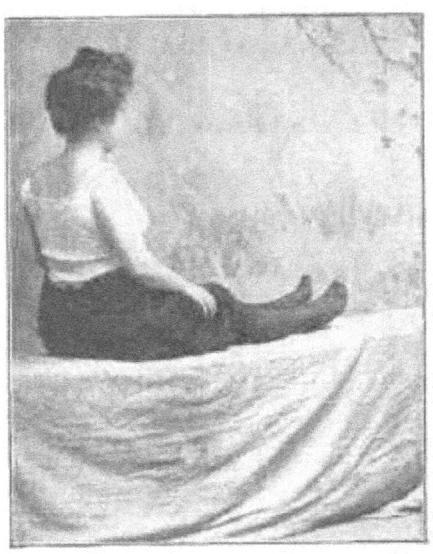

Exercise No. 18. Reclining on back and raising body to sitting position, as per illustration.

The choice of any special form of movement cure should be decided by the exigencies of their purpose to compensate the deficient opportunities of daily life. Persons engaged in sedentary occupations, alternating with domestic chances for arm exercise (wood-cutting, amateur carpentering, etc.,) should devote their leisure to pedestrianism or some class of gymnastics tending to develop the muscles of the lower motive organs. The great plurality of city dwellers who find daily occasion for walking matches against time, should give their arms the benefit of daily dumb-bell exercise, and patronize the flying trapeze on every visit to a public gymnasium.

A year's practice is almost sure to develop a prediction for some form of athletic exercise but the experience of every gymnasium teacher proves that, on the other hand, there are also individuals with a practically unconquerable aversion to special branches of his curriculum. These antipathies may often be founded on anomalies of physical structure, and are thus akin to the instinctive repugnance to certain kinds of food. Dr. W. Carpenter mentions the case of a boy who had a horror naturalis of mutton, and who at every attempt to overcome that dislike was seized with violent vomiting fits. His guardian was inclined to ascribe that caprice to the effects of imagination, and, by way of experiment, treated his ward to a meat-pie containing mutton disguised by spices, but the result remained the same, and the patient, who would have made a popular neighbor of certain Australian stock-farmers, was publicly recognized as a boy with a stomach that could not digest mutton.

And practice is almost equally unavailing to overcome the disinclination of some gymnasium pupils to special kinds of exercise—heel over head evolutions on a trapeze or horizontal bar, for instance. I have known gymnasts who complained of sick headaches whenever the routine of the educational programme obliged them to conquer that aversion, and a good rule in such cases is to accept the verdict of nature as final, if the repugnance should continue to assert itself after the tyro has mastered the technical difficulties of the exercise.

But it is also certain that habit develops an association of ideas between special ailments and their appropriate gymnastic remedies. I have mentioned the expedient of sailors who "work off" qualms of seasickness by volunteer exercise in the rigging and an old teacher of my acquaintance occasionally leaves the class-room to nip an incipient attack of asthma with a pair of dumbbells.

Hay-fever, I think, could often be knocked out with Indian clubs, and more than one victim of rheumatism has learned the trick of walking away from the premonitory symptoms of his affliction. A time may come when patients of all sorts will hurry to a gymnasium as they now hasten to a drug store.

The power of established prejudices, it is true, has almost no limits, but now and then yields to the dictates of fashion, and by good luck physical exercise is a cosmetic. People who do not realize that weakness and disease are crimes, may consent to recover because it is also the surest way to get pretty. They will appreciate the logic of their looking-glass.

"By their system of physical culture," says a Scotch author, "the Greeks realized that beautiful symmetry of shape which for us exists only in the ideal, or in the forms of divinity which they sculptured from figures of such perfect proportions."

Health is beauty; strength imparts ease of deportment; the paragons of fashion have constantly to recruit their ranks from the products of the forests and prairies; under the stimulus of outdoor exercise grace develops its fairest flowers

"Yet not one of all that did try Could play like Elfy, the Gypsy-boy."

Physical exercise is destined to effect the regeneration of the Caucasian race; but we should remember that it cannot at once counteract the mischief of all our manifold sins against the health laws of nature. It may prolong the lives of grog-drinking sailors, but cannot bleach their bottlenoses. It enables the hunters of the Pampas to digest a diet of bull-beef, but cannot save them from lung diseases if they pass the nights in smoky dug-outs.

Like the three Graces, the three remedies of Nature should go hand in hand.

Under the reign of old-time medical delusions, a sick man's first impulse was to "take something," i. c. to swallow a dose of poison drugs. A sanitarian's first thought, under the same circumstances, should be to stop swallowing, i. e. to fast for a day or two. Those who insist on "taking something" should be advised to take a cold bath, or an hour's exercise in the gymnasium.

Shall we dispense with chemical medicaments altogether?

The current of sanitary reform is certainly setting strongly in that very direction. In spite of quack-revivals, the time is coming and it not far, when intelligent physicians will prescribe drugs only for external application, as in cutaneous disorders, where their effect amounts to a direct removal of the cause, and internally only in analogous cases, as for the expulsion of intestinal parasites.

With these few exceptions, the disorders of the human organism will be trusted to the self-regulating tendency of nature, aided by the influence of the three natural stimulants: Fasting, Refrigeration, and Exercise. The disciples of Natural Hygiene will try to deserve the blessings which the dupes of the drug-monger attempt to buy across the counter; instead of changing their hospital or their course of medication they will change their habits, and their loss of faith in a few popular superstitions will be compensated by an abundant gain in health.

CHAPTER XVI

DETAILED ADVICE FOR TREATMENT

Wet sheet pack will be referred to in treatments advised and same can be taken as follows: Wet two heavy sheets in cold water: wring them out and lay them on a bed or sofa: let the patient lie on these, then take the top sheet and wrap tightly around the patient under the arms; then take the under sheet and wrap tightly around the patient over the arms. Of course this can be done with one sheet, but it is not quite so advantageous, as the \\et cloth does not come in contact with every part of the body. The patient should be allowed to remain there until the cloth is dry, or until he awakes, as it is quite usual for the patient to go to sleep under these circumstances.

Asthma:

Remain in the open air as much as possible. Be very careful to see that whenever indoors that the air is purified by thorough ventilation. Confine diet to two meals per day, though it would be far preferable if you would eat but one meal per day for at least one or two weeks. Take long walks in the open air, and acquire a habit of drawing in deep inhalations during these walks, expanding the lungs to their fullest capacity. While taking these breathing exercises make a habit of endeavoring to exhale every particle of air from the lungs that you can, and then inhale all that you possibly can. Use great care not to overeat. Every morning immediately upon arising, after taking sufficient exercise to accelerate the circulation thoroughly, take a cold sitz bath for one minute. Exercise numbers 7, 9, 10, 15 and 17 should be given especial attention, though the entire system could be used to advantage.

Bilious Fever:

Immediately upon appearance of the first symptoms take a wet sheet pack. Encourage the appetite for cold water, in every way, drinking copiously of same. Allow no food of any nature until the fever has diminished, and until there is strong appetite for same. Use cold sitz bath twice a day, and follow this each time with wet sheet pack until symptoms begin to disappear. The colon flushing treatment will sometimes hasten recovery in this complaint. As the symptoms begin to lessen in severity, some of the milder movements shown in preceding chapter can be taken with benefit.

Biliousness:

Confine the diet to one meal a day only. Eat very slowly. Encourage the appetite for fruits. Take long walks in the open air with many breathing exercises. Take the entire system of exercise as illustrated daily until slightly tired.

Blackheads:

Take up some thorough, systematic exercises for strengthening the entire organism, such as illustrated here. Take long walks in the open air, with many breathing exercises. Confine diet to two meals per day and be very careful to masticate the food thoroughly. Take two or three hot baths, with plenty of soap and water, per week. Apply hot and cold water alternately to the parts affected, at least twice a day. At night when retiring place a wet cloth on the affected parts so it will remain there until dry. Use a friction brush of some kind where the blackheads appear, once each day: this should lways precede the hot and cold applications. Bladder Disease:

Confine diet to one full meal or two light meals per day. Take long walks in the open air, with plenty of breathing exercises. Use only very pure water, and encourage your appetite in every way for this. If the disease is at all serious, all meats and stimulants of every character must be avoided.

Of the exercises here illustrated numbers 2, 3, 4, 8, 11, 13, 14 and 18 will be found especially beneficial, though the entire system should be used to a certain extent.

Blood Diseases:

Avoid all use of stimulants. Confine the diet to one meal per day for at least a week, though a longer continuance of same would be preferable. Take two or three hot baths per week, using plenty of soap. Take long walks in the open air, with deep breathing. If the skin is affected to any great extent, wet sheet pack will be found of advantage. Take the entire system of exercise as illustrated daily until slightly tired.

Boils:

If this trouble is chronic, one boil appearing after another, a general system of exercises and an abstemious diet for building up the general health is advised. Wet sheet pack will be found of advantage to open the pores of the skin and thus throw off impurities. Two or three hot baths per week, with plenty of soap, should always be taken, and great care should be used at meal times to thoroughly masticate every particle of food eaten. Deep breathing, and long walks will be found to advantage. There are two processes of treating boils: One is to "feed up" and thus more hurriedly bring the boil to a head, and another is, in case it is not too far advanced, to adopt a very abstemious diet and thus cause it to be absorbed into the circulation. If too far advanced, the former method is, of course, preferable.

Bright's Disease:

Same treatment as in Bladder Disease, though the necessity for the extreme abstemious diet is much stronger in this disease than in the other; in fact about the quickest way to cure a disease of this character is an absolute and protracted fast. By living very abstemiously, and avoiding all stimulants and meats the incipient phases of Bright's Disease can always be brought to a satisfactory cure. Bronchitis:

A cold sitz bath on arising. Wet sheet pack to follow same if symptoms are severe. One light meal a day until benefit is noticed. Deep breathing exercises, and great care to see that pure air is secured at all times.

Carbuncles:

Same treatment as for Boils.

Catarrh:

Treatment should aim at building up the general health, and purifying the blood in every way. Long walks and deep-breathing exercises in the open air. Regular use of some system of exercises such as are illustrated here. Every care to secure fresh air at all times, and special attention required to thorough mastication of food that digestion may be carried on more perfectly and more easily. The daily use of some antiseptic wash for the nostrils can be commended, such as a very mild solution of salt and water; about a quarter teaspoonful of salt to a glass of water. This solution must never be made stronger as it very often irritates the mucous membrane and makes the symptoms more severe if this mistake is made. Chicken-Pox:

Cold sitz bath and wet sheet pack twice a day. No food until symptoms begin to disappear, and strong appetite is noted.

Children's Diseases:

In all children's diseases the first, and about the most effective, remedy is to thoroughly flush the colon. Allow no food until there is a strong and unmistakable desire for same. Wet sheet pack can be advised once or twice a day in all fevers. Where there is severe pains in the bowels, apply very hot cloths, changing frequently.

131

Colds:

Stay in the open air as much as possible; long walks, and deep breathing will be found of advantage. A fast of a day or two will be found of great aid, and usually when the first meal is eaten after this fast but little will remain of the cold. Rubbing the skin until the circulation is thoroughly accelerated will be found of advantage. Treatment of hot steam baths can also be recommended in severe cases.

Constipation:

Exercise No. 8 will be found of special advantage in this particular complaint, and should be taken at least twice a day until thoroughly tired. Walking in the open air and deep breathing will also be found beneficial. In every case avoid white bread, eating whole wheat bread instead, and confine diet to two meals per day. An all-round system of exercises for building up the general system will also assist recovery. Consumption:

Remain in the open air as much as possible. Have the windows in your sleeping-room so arranged that the air in the inside contains the same amount of oxygen as that outside. Give especial attention to exercises numbers 1, 4, 5, 6, 7, 8, 9, 10, 12, 15, 16, 17 and 18. These exercises should be taken at least twice daily, and in the open air if possible making a habit during these exercises to draw in all the breath you can inhale. A long walk with deep breathing each day. The diet should be confined to one or two meals per day, and great care should be taken to thoroughly masticate each morsel. If symptoms are at all severe, the patient should retire at night in a wet sheet pack. The cure of this complaint will depend a great deal upon your ability to breathe pure air night and day, and upon your ability to secure a large amount of exercise

Coughs:

Long walks in the open air, and deep breathing will be found beneficial, also exercises numbers 1, 7, 15, 16 and 17. Great care should be taken not to overeat, and to thoroughly masticate every morsel. Confine diet to two meals

per day. Secure some pure, strained honey and use same frequently whenever cough becomes irritated. At night, upon retiring, wet cloth and wrap same around neck and chest and allow it to remain there until dry, or until morning.

Croup:

Wrap the throat and chest in cloths as hot as can possibly be borne; change same frequently until symptoms disappear.

Diabetes:

Same treatment as for Bladder Diseases and Bright's Disease.

Diarrhea:

A fast of a day or two would be the best manner of beginning treatment for this trouble, then confine diet to one meal a day; eat very slowly; masticate thoroughly; avoid meats and stimulants of all kinds. Eat Graham bread and vegetables, also fruits, if desired. Remain in the open air as much as possible.

Diphtheria:

Wet sheet pack should be given immediately upon appearance of the first symptoms; hot and cold cloths applied alternately around neck and chest previous to use of wet sheet pack. Colon flushing treatment should be given once or twice per clay; wet sheet pack twice a day; hot and cold applications to the throat as often as required. Encourage appetite for cold water, in every conceivable way.

Usually, the more \\ater than can be drunk, the better. Absolutely no food of any kind should be allowed until serious symptoms abate and until strong craving for food appears.

Dropsy:

One meal per day only. Eat but little meat. Take as much exercise in the open air as possible without serious fatigue. The entire system of exercises here illustrated will be found beneficial in this trouble, though exercises numbers 5, 6, 8, 10 and 12 can be especially recommended.

Dyspepsia:

One meal per day; masticate every morsel thoroughly. Avoid white bread, using Graham or rye bread instead. Never eat unless there is a strong desire for food. Every mouthful must be thoroughly enjoyed. The entire system of exercises illustrated in this book should be taken until slightly fatigued. Take long walks in the open air, and see that you breathe pure air at all times. Open the windows of your sleeping-room, both top and bottom, from six to twelve inches.

Eczema:

One meal per day. Avoid all meat and white bread. Take long walks in the open air, with plenty of deep breathing exercises. The entire system of exercises illustrated herewith once daily, taking each movement until slightly fatigued. One cold sitz bath daily, which should be followed by wet sheet pack.

Epilepsy:

One meal per day for the first week. Stay in the open air all you possibly can. Take all the exercises here illustrated, using each one until slightly fatigued. If symptoms are especially severe, wet sheet pack should be taken once daily.

Erysipelas:

Wet sheet pack upon the first appearance of the trouble. Fast until strong desire for food appears, then confine diet to one meal per day for a few days. Use exercises numbers 1, 7, 8, 9, 10, 11 and 15 after symptoms begin to disappear. Two or three times a day apply hot and cold cloths to the affected parts, alternating from one to the other.

Felons:

Same treatment as for Boils, though when they appear near the finger-nail, as is usual, if finger is dipped momentarily in water as hot as can be borne several times, they will sometimes be driven away and be absorbed by the circulation.

Gastric Fever:

Wet sheet pack immediately upon appearance of the symptoms, which should be followed or preceded by the colon flushing treatment. No food of any character until strong desire appears. Encourage the desire for cold water.

General Debility:

Each one of the exercises illustrated here should be taken, until slightly fatigued, once daily. The diet should be confined to one or two rneals per day. Great care should be taken to see that every morsel of food is thoroughly masticated. Live in the open air as much as possible, and a walk with deep breathing, each day until fatigued, will be found beneficial. Gout:

Avoid all meats and all stimulants. Confine diet to one meal per day. If pain is severe nothing should be eaten until it begins to subside. Bathe the affected parts once or twice daily in hot and cold water alternately, changing from one to the other.

Grippe:

If symptoms are severe, wet sheet pack and flushing colon treatment should be immediately taken. Absolutely no food until very strong desire for same appears. Be careful that very pure air be secured at all times. As the more severe symptoms disappear, the system of exercises herewith illustrated can be taken with advantage.

Headache:

Encourage desire for hot water all you can. If convenient, take steam vapor bath. Eat no foods except some light fruit until symptoms disappear. The flushing of the colon treatment in very many cases affords almost immediate relief. Great care should be taken that fresh, pure air is secured at all times, in fact severe headache is very often caused by simply breathing bad air.

Heart Disease:

Take exercises numbers I, 4, 5, 6, 7, 8, 9, 10, 12 and 13 once daily, continuing same until slightly fatigued. Take a long walk each day, with many deep-breathing exercises. Confine the diet to two light meals or one full meal per clay. Thoroughly masticate every morsel of food eaten. This process will strengthen the heart, though immediate satisfactory results must not be expected.

Hemorrhoids:

Cold sitz bath after accelerating circulation, with exercise upon arising each morning. Until symptoms begin to disappear only one meal a day should be eaten, and food should be masticated very thoroughly; but little meat should be eaten. Unless symptoms are severe, long walks with deep-breathing exercises, will be found of advantage. If especially severe, the flushing of the colon treatment can sometimes be recommended.

Indigestion:

Same treatment as for Dyspepsia. Don't eat until very hungry.

Insomnia:

Treatment for this trouble should be constitutional. The entire system of exercises illustrated here should be taken once daily. Long walks in the open air, with deep breathing, can also be commended. The diet should be confined to not more than two meals a day, and great care should be taken not to overeat. At the last meal it would be advisable to eat freely of lettuce, dressed with oil and lemon-juice, with salt to taste.

Jaundice:

Same treatment as for Biliousness.

Kidney Disease:

Same treatment as in Bladder Diseases.

Liver Disease:

Same treatment as for Biliousness.

Lumbago:

Take exercises numbers I, 2, 4, 5, 6, 12, 14, 16 and 17. Apply hot and cold cloths alternately to the affected parts twice per day, until the severe symptoms begin to disappear. Be careful not to overeat, and confine diet to one or two meals per day, masticating very thoroughly. Malaria:

Treatment for this trouble simply requires a course for building up the general health. The entire system of exercises here illustrated should be taken daily, each movement being continued until slightly fatigued. Long walks in the open air are advisable, unless too weak, though pure air should be procured at all times. A sitz bath, followed by a wet sheet pack, taken daily, will be found of advantage.

Measles:

Immediately upon appearance of first symptoms give a wet sheet pack, followed or preceded by the colon flushing treatment. Wet sheet pack to be continued two or three times a day until symptoms disappear. No food of any kind should be given until a strong desire for same appears, and the desire for water should be encouraged in every way.

Nervous Debility:

Same treatment as for General Debility.

Neuralgia:

Apply hot and cold cloths to the affected parts, alternating from one to the other. Encourage drinking of hot and cold water all you can. Wet sheet pack will be found of advantage if convenient. No food should be eaten until strong desire for same appears.

Palpitation:

Same treatment as for Heart Disease.

Pneumonia:

Wet sheet pack, followed or preceded by colon flushing treatment. Wet sheet pack should be given two or three times per day. No food of any character should be allowed until serious symptoms abate. Encourage the desire to drink large quantities of water. As soon as the more serious symptoms abate, the exercises numbers I, 7, 9, 15, 16 and 17 can be used to advantage. Great care should be taken to secure perfectly pure air at all times in this trouble, as patients suffering from this disease often die from this one neglect.

Rheumatism:

Wet sheet pack twice a day. One meal a day for the first week. Meats of all kinds should be avoided: food should be very thoroughly masticated. Massage will be found beneficial. One or two-day fast will hasten recovery. Salt

138

Rheum:

Same treatment as for Eczema.

Sciatica:

Exercises numbers 2, 3, 8, 9, 10, 11, 14 and 18 should be taken twice daily until slightly fatigued. Exercise No. 2 should be given especial attention. Confine diet to two meals per day, and eat very slowly. At night, upon retiring, apply a wet cloth to the affected parts.

Scrofula:

Same treatment as for Blood Diseases.

Skin Diseases:

Same treatment as for Blood Diseases.

Sore Throat:

Same treatment as for Bronchitis.

Typhoid Fever:

Same treatment as Gastric Fever.

Whooping Cough:

Same treatment as for Croup.